Praise for *The P...*

"A helpful book on sin...
mind."

— Gerald G. Jampolsky, MD, author of
Love Is Letting Go of Fear

"I love this book. It is clear, original, interesting, welcoming, and above all, helpful. I can't imagine anyone who would not benefit from reading even a small part of it. I especially like the deeper understanding Blake brings to the subject of prayer within a book on meditation."

— Hugh Prather, author of
How to Live in the World and Still Be Happy

"This wise book grounds the reader in the great meditative traditions while offering a clear framework for practicing in today's busy world. Tobin Blake does more than just point out the path to serenity; he is a knowledgeable guide to the points of interest and the pitfalls along the way."

— Patricia Monaghan, coauthor of
Meditation: The Complete Guide

"There is a revelation in stillness; it opens us to the Divine, and expands our awareness. Meditation is really an open secret and the most precious of spiritual practices. Tobin Blake understands the meaning of stillness and has learned it through his own meditation experience. As practical as it is profound, *The Power of Stillness* is an effective evocation of the desire to sit, to just be."

— Wayne Teasdale, author of *The Mystic Heart*

everyday
meditation

everyday
meditation

100 DAILY MEDITATIONS
for Health, Stress Relief, and Everyday Joy

Tobin Blake

New World Library
Novato, California

New World Library
14 Pamaron Way
Novato, California 94949

Text design by Tona Pearce Myers

Library of Congress Cataloging-in-Publication Data
Blake, Tobin, date.
Everyday meditation : 100 daily meditations for health, stress relief, and everyday joy / Tobin Blake.
   p.   cm.
Includes bibliographical references (p. 267).
ISBN 978-1-60868-060-3 (pbk. : alk. paper)
1. Meditation. 2. Meditations. I. Title.
BL627.B554 2012
158.1'2—dc23   2011041009

First printing, February 2012
ISBN 978-1-60868-060-3
Printed in Canada on 100% postconsumer-waste recycled paper

New World Library is a proud member of the Green Press Initiative.

10 9 8 7 6 5 4 3 2

*This book is dedicated with eternal gratitude
to my mother,*

*Frances Joan Dresser
(October 16, 1937–July 10, 2004),*

who taught me the power of unconditional love —

forever a graceful soul.

Contents

Part One: Understanding Meditation

Introduction..3
Meditation 101...13

Part Two: Developing Your Technique

Daily Meditations: Day 1–Day 10.............................25
Overcoming Obstacles: Day 11–Day 20...................43
The Development of Peace: Day 21–Day 30............67

Part Three: Reprogramming the Waterfall

Introduction..93
Opening to the Mystical Moment: Day 31–Day 40...................95
The Key to Emotional Balance: Day 41–Day 50......................119
The Law of Reciprocity: Day 51–Day 60..............................147
The *Real* Justification for Forgiveness: Day 61–Day 70..........169
Health and Healing: Day 71–Day 80.....................................193

Healing Relationships and Sexuality: Day 81–Day 90..............213
Developing a Daily Practice: Day 91–Day 100.......................237

Epilogue: Connecting with Your Inner Teacher......................261
Notes..267
About the Author..269

PART ONE

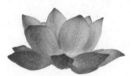

UNDERSTANDING
MEDITATION

Introduction

One day when I was first learning meditation, I stood on the rear porch of my father's home overlooking Oregon's looping McKenzie River and watched as the sun faded over the mountains to the west. While I was growing up in Los Angeles, the city felt like a vast, hardened prison from which no escape seemed possible. Back then, my only moments of release came while gazing across the Pacific Ocean, where humans and their works ended, and nature and hers began — toward the freedom of the open horizon.

Likewise, here was the grand McKenzie River, carving its course with no mind for people, time, or obstacles of any type. Set a mountain in front of this river, and it would chew the mountain into a valley. I appreciate that spirit! At the time, I did not realize what enchanted my eye so, but now I know what it was. It was not the beauty of the land, the sweep of the river, or the sunset. It was the freedom of the moment that hooked me. For just one instant, I lost myself to life's flow and experienced a peace unlike any I had felt before.

You have probably had moments like this too, when you have "lost yourself" and perhaps even felt touched by some mysterious, magnetic force that seemed to connect with your own life from somewhere deep within. For most people, these moments are like glimpses through a window that is ordinarily hidden but that serves to remind us that there is far more to life than what we can see, touch, or hear. They are mystical moments that, in a flash, infuse life with meaning and a renewed sense of purpose.

The practice of meditation is the practice of actively making yourself open to this experience and the far more compelling states that can follow, for this common, passing experience is only the tip of the iceberg when it comes to inner space. Practiced actively, meditation can lead to states of sublime peace and profound joy that are so powerful, they defy description. Hindus, who have been meditating for thousands of years, refer to these ecstatic meditative states as *samadhi*. During meditation, you switch your focus from the external world — with its complexity, constant stress, and sense of separation — toward the internal world, which is the opposite in every respect. Through this shift you may discover that just beyond our ordinary human awareness, life is a vast, interconnected network that exists in a state of peaceful union. Essentially, through meditation you learn that you are not a physical being living a temporary life of separation from the rest of the world, but a spirit living an eternal life of union with every living creature in the universe. You are a part of them, and they are a part of you.

This realization is impossible to describe because there is no parallel experience in the world to compare it to, making it doubly difficult to understand intellectually. Deep meditation has been likened to orgasm, but I think this analogy is misleading. Rather, I would say it is akin to the instant immediately *preceding* the release of orgasm, except that it never ceases to build in intensity and depth, and the experience has a certain purity and innocence that sex does not. After twenty years of devoted meditation, I am still wondering how deep the rabbit hole goes. I am gradually coming to believe that to be in tune with Spirit is to be in tune with an ever-expanding creative impulse to forever let go, to forever give oneself away. As for the sensations this expansive impulse creates, if the mainstream populace suspected the kind of intense joy that meditation can trigger, people would be knocking down the doors of their local meditation center to learn its secrets. It's no wonder that the practice has proved so effective at promoting health and healing. Happiness and peace boost the immune system naturally.

This book is set up to do more than merely introduce you to the practice of meditation on a theoretical level. It has been divided into three sections. Part 1, "Understanding Meditation," will acquaint you with all the essential ABCs of meditative practice, and will help you understand what meditation is and how you can use it to live a happier, healthier life. Part 2, "Developing Your Technique," consists of the first thirty exercises of the hundred-day journey that forms the backbone of this book. This section will give you a thorough, hands-on introduction to the world's major meditative techniques, allowing you to discover the joys of the practice firsthand. There is really no other way to learn meditation. And if you already meditate, the exercises will help you to diversify your practice and take it to the next level.

Although meditation is easy enough in theory, without the right tools it can seem to be just the opposite. Many people who begin meditation give up before realizing all it can offer them. This is because there can be tremendous psychological resistance at first. Many meditation teachings instruct students only in the bare techniques, such as mantra, zazen, mindfulness, and visualization, and offer very little help in overcoming the obstacles to deep meditative states. This book is different. While it *does* teach the ABCs and techniques, part 3, "Reprogramming the Waterfall," will take you beyond the forms of meditation and help you release your own psychological resistance so that you can develop a deep and lasting meditative practice.

Together, the three sections of this book provide a hands-on experiential journey into the meditative experience, as well as presenting a spiritual mind-training system for living a more conscious, peace-filled life. The system focuses on three primary objectives:

1. *Daily practice.* This may seem obvious, but you might be surprised by how many people believe they can get something by reading books about meditation without ever actually trying it. Take my word on this point up front — *you can't*! You do have to meditate, and regularly, to benefit from it. The good news is that the benefits are incredible. In fact, meditation is one of the very best things you can do to improve both your physical and psychological health. It's right up there with quitting smoking. The trick is, just like with exercise, you have to do it. This is an active book that contains one hundred daily meditations to help you take this step. Think of these hundred days as a journey of self-discovery that has been set up not only to get you meditating but also to assist you in rooting out and healing the hurts and fears you have accumulated over many years. Doing so will bring you peace and increase the power of your meditative experiences many times over.

2. *Understand and deal with the resistance.* To achieve deep meditative states, you will have to uncover the things that hold you back. We all have some resistance to meditation. As you press toward the center of your being, which is the direction of meditation, you will have to work your way through many layers of resistance. This is what makes meditation feel like work — and make no mistake, *it is work.* It is self-work of the highest order: conscious *personal development.* By learning how to meditate, you are embarking on a powerful journey of healing unlike anything else in the world. Meditation takes you inward, directly into contact with your core self (spirit) — an experience that is purifying, empowering, and often exhilarating. An incredible power flows from core self, and

aligning yourself with it can change your life in an instant. We'll talk more about core self later. For now, you need to know that besides getting you to practice meditation daily, this book is designed to assist you in the process of uncovering the root causes behind your natural resistance to meditation.

3. *Reprogram the waterfall.* If you already meditate, you are no doubt familiar with the endless stream of thoughts that runs in the background of your mind. This stream of *word stuff* is so constant that Buddhists call it the "waterfall of thought" because the sound is as steady as the drone of a roaring waterfall — endless and deafening. When you first start meditating, it may even seem as if your thoughts are speeding up; however, this is not the case. You are only becoming more aware of the constant activity of thought. Some people try to force discipline upon their thoughts, but this is rarely successful. You cannot shut down the waterfall of *thought stuff*. However, you *can* change its content. Most people's thoughts are substantially composed of negative programming — the products of unhealed guilt, fear, and anger. Such emotions are inherently antithetical to peace, which is the state of meditation. Therefore, negative thoughts make meditation difficult. To deepen your meditations, it is vital to change the background thoughts of your mind to reflect gentleness and other positive emotions. The one hundred meditations that follow are designed to help you begin this process of reprogramming. In a sense, this book is not only about meditation; it is also a course in mind training. Reprogramming your inner dialogue will help you in other ways besides improving your meditative practice. By exchanging a negative waterfall of thought for a positive one, you will see how your whole life can be transformed, for negative thoughts not only

interfere with meditative practice but also affect everything in our lives, including our health, happiness, and
relationships.

There are many great reasons to meditate. Modern science
has been exploring meditation for decades, and what it has found
is startling. Some things are obvious: During meditation, blood
pressure and heart rate decrease, respiration slows, and alpha
wave activity in the brain increases (indicating a peaceful state).
In general, stress levels drop, an effect that alone could save con-
sumers billions of dollars in health care costs annually. Some es-
timates suggest that over 90 percent of doctor visits are linked to
unmanaged stress.

Besides the more generic effect of stress relief, it has been
discovered that meditation also produces physical changes in the
body. In one study, published in the journal *NeuroImage*, a group
of UCLA researchers discovered that the hippocampus and areas
within the orbito-frontal cortex of meditators were enlarged, indicating that the brain is *physically* affected by the practice. Talk about
expanding your mind! The cortex is associated with higher human
functions like decision making, positive emotion, and memory.

Other recent groundbreaking research delved even deeper
into the biological effects of regular meditation. In collabora-
tion with the Genomics Center at Beth Israel Deaconess Medi-
cal Center, researchers at the Benson-Henry Institute for Mind
Body Medicine at Massachusetts General Hospital discovered that
meditation reaches straight to the root of our biological programming — our genes themselves. They reported significant
differences in the expressions of more than 2,200 genes between
meditators and nonmeditators. Some of these genes included
those responsible for inflammation, the handling of free radi-
cals, and programmed cell death, three killers that act as Father
Time's right-hand henchmen when it comes to aging and disease.
Herbert Benson, MD, the center's director, said of the findings,

"Now we've found how changing the activity of the mind can alter the way basic genetic instructions are implemented." This is a powerful statement. For many years, researchers have pondered meditation's extraordinary healing effects, which were easily detectable through rudimentary experiments. Now we are finally digging below the surface effects of meditation and uncovering some of the deeper causes behind the physical health benefits. Somehow, meditation is reshaping the very building blocks of our bodies.

The horizon of emerging meditation research appears to be no less promising. We are learning more every day. For instance, in an interview on the national radio show *Speaking of Faith*, Doris Taylor, MD, cited preliminary research into meditation's incredible effect on stem cells. Taylor is a cardiac researcher best known for resurrecting the dead heart of a rat by injecting it with stem cells. These cells are now considered one of the primary keys to aging and disease. Basically, as our stem cells die off, we age, and stress literally destroys these cells. When it comes to slowing aging, then, stem cells are genetic gold. In essence, the younger your stem cells are, the younger, biologically speaking, you are. Meditation may be doing a couple of things here. For one, it slows the process of stem cell aging simply by alleviating stress; however, there appears to be more to the story than that. It turns out that meditation may increase the number of stem cells in the blood. During a preliminary study at the University of Wisconsin, researchers noted a significant spike in the number of stem cells in the bloodstream of an experienced meditator after just fifteen minutes of practice. Mind you, this was not a well-controlled, double-blind study meant for publication, but a casual investigation by a group of curious scientists. That said, the results were stunning. During the interview, Taylor, who was barely able to conceal her excitement, called it "the largest increase [of stem cells] I've ever seen."

This may help explain some of meditation's major impacts on our health. Regular practitioners can expect the following:

- A 33 percent decrease in the chance of stroke

- A 50 percent decrease in overall cancer rates

- A decrease of up to 80 percent in the rate of heart disease
  — America's number one killer of both men and women

No medication currently on the market shows such remarkable and widespread healing effects, and this is to say nothing of the psychological benefits of the practice. While meditation is clearly good for the body, it's also great for the mind. People who meditate regularly report a greater overall sense of satisfaction with their lives and relationships, and lower incidence and severity of depression, anxiety, and panic attacks. This translates to real life as less pain and more joy. Simply put, meditation is the very best of natural medicine, and it has absolutely no negative side effects.

It's rare that anything in this world can offer so much and yet cost so little. In fact, there is no direct cost. To achieve the results that will lead you to a happier, healthier life, all that is needed is consistency. Your practice doesn't need to be perfect. Just do it, every day.

Beyond committing to regular practice, the most helpful attitude is to regard meditation as an unfolding journey that involves expanding your consciousness away from ego-centered awareness and toward Spirit-centered awareness. This is a gentle progression. Have patience and trust the process. During meditation, you close your eyes and turn your attention inward, away from the world and toward the inner landscape of your life, your mind, and ultimately your core self. It is during this sacred communion with your true self, which exists in a state of peace at the center of your being — independent of ego, personality, and your body — that you begin to heal your inner wounds and grow in the most profound sense of the word. In this respect, the journey of meditation is the most sacred journey any of us could make. It is a journey of healing — of coming to peace with the world, our relationships, and ultimately ourselves. By communing with our core self, we are simultaneously connecting with the unfathomable Source energy that is the creative force behind every heartbeat, every breath, and every living atom of the universe.

Pause and reflect on this. *Meditation reconnects you consciously with the energy that brought all life into being.* Our connection with Source has never been broken. We could not live without it. However, most people are completely unaware that this connection even exists. Meditation can be thought of as an exercise that cleans and polishes your link to Source. This is what makes it such a profound healing practice. Through this ancient, time-honored exercise, you are literally attempting to connect, in full awareness, with the Power that brought all life into existence, both physical and nonphysical — the galaxies and planets; the countless stars that light our night sky; the billions of people, animals, and insects that populate our world and all the others; and every cell that makes up your own body. The magnitude of creation is impossible to grasp from a human perspective, but as you align yourself with Source, its life-giving energy flows through you — healing you at every level and infusing you with a sense of new life and new purpose. This energy is already a part of you. All you need to do is learn how to release the inner blocks that keep you unaware of it.

Meditation 101

magine yourself walking along a garden path toward a brilliant light that brings warmth and nourishment to everything it shines upon. The path is open and the way gentle, flanked by gardens brimming with life. This is a peaceful, safe place, beautiful to gaze upon.

If you turn around and look behind you, however — back the way you came from — the light is no longer perceived directly. Instead, it is positioned at your back, and suddenly the change in your own positioning casts the world into shadow. Now, the shadows are nothing more than a play of light and darkness, but in them reality — and the beauty of your natural surroundings — is cloaked; and as you gaze upon the shifting darkness, you are left to the whim of your imagination. In a world of shadows, you could see anything, pleasant or ghoulish, but either way, it would not be real. It would be merely a reflection of your own thoughts, fears, and beliefs. In essence, it would be a projection of your mind.

When it comes to the world we perceive outside of us, this analogy is not far from the truth. When you look out and upon the external world, you are turning and facing away from the great Source of life. Life did not manifest from the outside in, but from the inside out. By focusing on the external, then, you put yourself in a position in which what you perceive is so heavily influenced by your own state of mind that the reality of the world is blotted out.

Meditation is the conscious act of turning around and facing the other way — inward. For just a little while each day, you sit down, close your eyes to the outside world, and turn your attention toward the inside world, where your core self, which is a direct extension of Source, still exists. The *core self* is the original creative spark from which grew everything in your life as you know it. To use an analogy, *it is the foundation upon which your home is built.* Everyone has a core self, although they may call it by other names, such as *soul* or *spirit*. I prefer to use the expression *core self* only because it is more descriptive, and also it does not have the negative connotations of more traditional terms. This is the same reason why I prefer to use the word *Source* more often than *God*, although these words are also interchangeable.

Your core self exists in a pure state of being, beyond every self-concept you hold, all beliefs, your individual thoughts and mind, your physical body, and even the passage of time. Consider the consciousness of infants before they have had time to develop biases; labels; self-concepts; ambitions; thoughts about what is right and wrong, large and small, pretty and ugly, good and bad, short and tall; and so on. They may quickly develop a weak ego, but they are far freer than most adults. Infants live in a world of purified existence, in which they fulfill the role of being an infant without question. As a result, most infants are more in tune with their core self than are adults. I believe this is the reason why Jesus told his followers that they must become "like little children" in order to enter Heaven. It is also the reason why infants can be so enchanting, why their eyes sparkle with life, and why their laughter fills the heart with joy. It is also the reason why their crying and their tears can be so incredibly painful for adults. When an infant cries, it is like the sound of God crying. We can barely stand it.

Most of the things, ideas, personality traits, and thoughts we think of as making up our lives are not really life at all. They are just *stuff* that has been added on to the core self — that bare, essential energy of life that infants are so in tune with. Everything else is ego, also known as the *false self*, which then becomes identified with the body and the external world. You are more than this.

Think of a deciduous tree with its roots, trunk, and branches. These are like the core self. Year after year, these parts of the tree do not change much. The flowers and leaves, on the other hand, may bloom and grow, but come autumn, they change color and spin to the ground, only to be replaced by a new generation of leaves and flowers when spring arrives. One of the problems with our lives is that we have become transfixed with the changing properties of life on earth — the changing states of ego and the physical body. When you reach down into your depths, you are attempting to release all this extra stuff, if only temporarily, so that you can come into direct, conscious contact with your core. Essentially, you are attempting to liberate your attention from the pattern of changing leaves and trying to sense your oneness with the Tree of Life itself.

While it may not seem to be this way at first, shifting your focus toward the core self is the most natural direction of your mind. It takes a great deal of energy to maintain an external focus — so much, in fact, that doing so exhausts us to the point that we are forced into a state of unconsciousness every night. The moment you lie down in your bed at night and free your attention, you go speeding inward into the realm of "sleep," which is really nothing more than an *unconscious* sojourn into inner space and core self. This union with core self is what makes sleep so important for both mental and physical health, even though it lacks the full power of conscious contact with core self. It is still healing and refreshing. Meditation takes you into these same inner territories, except it does so while you are fully awake and aware.

How to Meditate

When you close your eyes, what do you see? It may have occurred to you by now that you have closed your eyes many times before and experienced little of interest. Most people see their inner mind as nothing more than a field of darkness overlaid by the constant sound of their inner dialogue. This stream of thoughts is what I referred to in the introduction as the "waterfall of thought." We all have one, and it is just this wall of thoughts that keeps us trapped inside the narrow sphere of our own heads, identified with ego. As your thoughts grow more peaceful and quiet, it becomes easy to sense your connection with core self.

Initially, you may or may not view meditation as a means to find your core self, and there is no reason to do so in order to benefit from the practice. Perhaps you are interested in meditation only for stress relief, to improve your health, or for other reasons. In any case, you will find that the practice still requires you to contend with your own thoughts, and in fact this is one of the primary focuses of most techniques. Many meditative practices consist of focusing on a simple sentence, word, or image, essentially a single "thought," to the exclusion of everything else. The idea is to keep the mind focused on one thing or practice while doing your best to avoid interrupting thought patterns that trap your attention and steer you away from the meditation. In this way, the practitioner is better able to sense and connect with the quiet sphere of peace that can be felt between thoughts, beyond the waterfall.

There are many specific techniques for achieving this. Zazen, for instance, is a popular Zen practice that focuses on becoming *mindful of* (essentially, paying attention to) a particular sensation, such as the feeling of your breath entering and exiting your body. Sometimes, however, zazen practices may suggest specific concentration exercises, like counting the breaths. For example, when you breathe in, you count that as "*one*" (to yourself, silently). Then, as you exhale, you think "*two*." Inhale, "*three*." Exhale, "*four*," and so on. The object of this exercise is to count your breaths without allowing your mind to drift from the practice. Anytime you find that you have stopped counting and started thinking, you gently but firmly redirect your mind back to the practice of counting your breaths, starting again with "one."

This form of zazen is closely related to another popular form of meditation known as *mantra*. Instead of counting the breaths, however, mantra uses a single word, sound, or short sentence as the primary focus, to be repeated throughout the meditation either out loud or silently to oneself. Once again, the idea is to concentrate on the mantra instead of other thoughts. The mantra may be timed to coincide with the respiratory cycle, as in zazen, or not.

Both of these techniques may be good choices for people with a very structured mind but not as good for people with an active imagination. For those who prefer to use imagery, *guided* meditations and other *visualization* practices often prove the right fit. Visualization typically involves focusing on a predetermined image, which could be just about anything. You might, for instance, imagine yourself meditating on the beach while trying to sense your unity with the ocean; or you could picture the image of a deity, a candle and its flame, a pebble, a temple, a flower, formless light — you get the idea. As with other styles of meditative practice, the object is to stay centered on the visualization while allowing other thoughts to pass through your mind without pulling your attention away.

In *chakra* meditation, practice typically involves the attempt to hold your attention on energy vortices that are thought to bridge the subtle spiritual and gross physical bodies. One such practice is *third eye* meditation. This type of meditative practice may be difficult to understand unless you try it out, because the instructions often consist of vague suggestions like "Keep your attention focused at the point between the eyebrows." Chakra meditation is a style that lies somewhere between very structured practices, such as counting the breath, and significantly less structured teachings, like *just sitting*, which is a technique that offers virtually no guidance other than to suggest that practitioners sit quietly and allow their thoughts to come and go without any personal involvement with them.

As you can see, what most meditation techniques have in common is that the meditator concentrates on a specific word, sentence, image, or practice (like counting the breaths or minding a feeling), to the exclusion of other thoughts. All such techniques are effective to some degree because turning inward is actually quite natural. Therefore, the simple act of *trying* to change the direction of your focus will always succeed to some degree. Yet, as I have already suggested, techniques alone are somewhat limited in themselves. The reason for this is that they focus primarily on the *form* of practice and don't address the psychological obstacles that hold students back from getting the most from their efforts. When you give students a mantra to repeat and tell them to keep their mind focused on it, doing so inevitably proves extremely difficult and quite often serves only to frustrate them. This is particularly true when they've received no other spiritual training.

Here, I am defining *spiritual training* as teachings intended to help students release fear and bring their mind to a state of peace, which is the key to deep meditation. This is why, as you will notice, the one hundred daily meditations in this book teach more than just the techniques of meditation. As they progress, they increasingly focus on helping you to retrain your thoughts — or, as I like to say, reprogram your waterfall.

How Long to Meditate

Well-meaning meditation instructors often make a serious blunder by suggesting that students spend excessive amounts of time meditating. This is a mistake that has gone on long enough, and it reflects the typically American misperception that bigger is better, more is *more valuable*, and excess is success. Long meditations only increase fatigue in most beginning students and may, as a result, add to resistance. Meditation doesn't require much time at all. Anybody can close their eyes and spend an hour or longer thinking. This is not meditation. In contrast, just one instant of focused meditation is enough to make a deep inner connection. Your core self is not far away. It's a part of you. In fact, it's the only real part of you. Everything else is just temporary stuff, like clouds drifting across the sky. How long, then, does it take to connect to your core self? As will be discussed later, it doesn't take any time at all. What it does require is pure desire and simple freedom from conflict.

Therefore, as you proceed, please keep in mind that the quality of your practicing is much more important than the quantity. Instead of meditating for extended periods of time, if you want to spend more time on your practice, I suggest you increase the number of daily sessions. For instance, if you plan on spending thirty minutes a day meditating, instead of doing one thirty-minute meditation, try three ten-minute meditations — morning, afternoon, and evening. Or two fifteen-minute sittings. Of course, it's fine for those with more experience to sit for however long feels pleasant. For some, sessions of thirty to sixty minutes may be appropriate. For students who are brand new to the practice, anywhere from five to twenty minutes is certainly adequate.

How to Sit

I want you to keep two words in mind while deciding how to sit during meditation: *comfortable* and *proud*. While there are a number of specific positions — such as the famous lotus position, in which you sit cross-legged with one or both ankles over the opposite thigh(s) — how you sit during meditation is not all that important. There are, however, a few points to keep in mind regarding posture and position.

1. *Get comfortable:* First and foremost, you should sit in a way that makes you feel comfortable and at ease. You

may sit in a chair, on a bed, or on a sofa, with your legs crossed or your feet flat on the floor; or you can adopt a cross-legged position on the floor. Use pillows to adjust your position and provide support and comfort.

2. *Be proud:* Do not lie down, which increases withdrawal, a tendency that can be problematic during meditation. Instead, sit up tall and proud, which will help keep you energized and will curtail excess tension that can arise from slouching. Keep your back comfortably straight, with your head up and shoulders erect. Rest your hands in your lap or on your legs, wherever they fall naturally, and above all else, *relax.* Attempt to gain a sense of your muscles loosening up, and let any tension and stress drain away. Give yourself permission to just let it all go and be at peace for a while — in body and in mind.

Other than following these simple guidelines, forget about your body while you practice. With the exception of a few techniques, meditation is a shift away from the bodily level, and obsessing about how to sit, where to place this or that body part, what to do with your hands, and so on is just one more distraction from the practice itself.

With these basics in mind, the most helpful attitude when learning meditation is one of nonjudgment. Do not judge the experiences you have on a day-to-day basis, whether they seem good or bad at the time. Meditation is an evolution that gently expands your consciousness over time, but along the way you will go through many stages of expansion and contraction. What this means is, you will experience stages of deepening meditative awareness followed by times during which your meditations will seem to become shallower. This is a natural process, but the overall direction is always one of growth. Retrogression is temporary and, in fact, important. These alternating periods of growth and retreat produce a waxing and waning effect that provides the ultimate contrast between being at peace and in sync with core self, and then losing touch. Through these contrasting stages, you will learn which direction brings peace and which discomfort, and thus you will develop the necessary motivation for going deeper into your meditations. Without this, the journey would quickly become stagnant.

So don't judge. Your only "job" is to focus on your daily practice and let the meditative journey unfold naturally.

Another helpful attitude is to approach your practicing with a feeling of deep reverence. Don't just plop down to practice, but pause for a moment before you sit down, and remind yourself of the importance of what you are doing. You are trying to reach beyond your body, beyond images and thoughts, and even past the world itself, directly into your core. You are seeking direct conscious experience of the original spark of life that exists at the center of your being and that connects you directly with Source. Touching your core, even if for only an instant, is an experience of indescribable power. It is so compelling that once you have felt it in full awareness, your entire life will shift in a bold new direction — toward peace, toward authentic power, and toward healing at the most profound level.

PART TWO

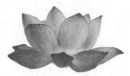

DEVELOPING YOUR TECHNIQUE

Daily Meditations

The following one hundred daily meditations are designed to help you develop a rich and vibrant meditation practice or, for experienced meditators, to increase the depth of your current practice. Specific instructions will be given as you proceed. Use only one meditation per day. If you find particular exercises especially enjoyable, however, by all means use them for several days in a row if you like. Just be certain to continue through the remainder of the exercises when you are ready. For best results, do not skip days, and at a minimum, be sure to read through everything. Each lesson includes important tips for your success.

The daily meditations are interlaced with short chapters that discuss a variety of topics related to meditation. Read through and carefully consider these before you proceed with the next daily meditation. You may wish to refer back to these chapters as needed.

To get the most out of the exercises, I recommend that you meditate twice each day, once in the morning and once at night, for as long as you feel comfortable. If you cannot make time twice a day, at least endeavor to set aside a few minutes each day. Another important point here is that if you miss full days, or even weeks, don't use the lapse as an excuse to quit altogether. As soon as you are willing and able, pick up again right where you left off. You will probably encounter some ego resistance to meditation early on. Be prepared for this. The one hundred daily meditations will help you to understand this resistance and work through it, but you still have to do your part.

Beginners should probably aim to meditate between five and twenty minutes per session, while more advanced students may choose to meditate for up to an hour or more. However, regardless of how long you practice, try to give each meditation your total focus, doing your best to set aside everything else that's going on in your life for just a short period of time. As noted previously, when it comes to meditation, longer is not necessarily better. It isn't particularly helpful to sit for long periods of time if you are not really concentrating; therefore, you will probably find shorter, concentrated meditations more beneficial.

While meditating, if you experience anxiety that does not go away after a few minutes, open your eyes until the feeling dissipates and then resume your practice. If it persists, end your practice until it is time for your next meditation. Most anxiety is minimal and easily passes by as the peace beyond it becomes increasingly compelling. Like most distractions in meditation, if you don't make a big deal out of it, it will disappear on its own.

The first thirty days of our journey together will walk you through a series of exercises that will get you practicing regularly and help you to discover which techniques are most effective for you. The remaining meditations will be increasingly concerned with the development of inner peace and reprogramming the waterfall of thought. They will feature daily thoughts for reflection and contemplation to be used in conjunction with whatever style of meditation you've come to prefer. These daily thoughts can also be used at any time during the day to help you maintain a positive, tranquil mindset. This will be discussed further in part 3.

Just remember, meditation is the highest sort of work; therefore, if it feels difficult at first, so be it. Meditation will challenge you to grow in the most profound ways, and this does require effort.

However, rapid success is also quite possible. Some people take to meditative practice right away. Whatever is the case for you, take one day at a time, one practice at a time. Give some thought to each day's meditation, and do your best with the exercises. Nothing more is needed. Meditation is like a high-interest investment account. A little effort yields large returns over time. Look at these exercises as times set aside for you to destress and unwind, and to begin living a more conscious, inspired, and balanced life.

Day 1

We are going to begin our hundred-day journey together with a simple exercise. The meditation for today is a form of zazen, already briefly discussed. If you are just trying meditation for the first time, it may seem more like an exercise in futility than anything else, but I promise you that there is a point to it. Try not to judge any of the meditations that follow, but simply practice them to the best of your ability. We are not so much concerned with the specific meditative practices as with the state of mind they lead to.

If this, or any other practice, seems a bit pointless, keep in mind that the simplest meditations are often the most effective. Ideally, we want to use techniques that are not overly complex so that we can gain a sense of the internal peace that lies *beyond* the meditative procedure. Using heavy, complicated meditations is like overspicing a meal. Delicate flavors can easily be ruined by a heavy-handed chef.

1. Two times today, morning and evening, find a quiet space where you can be alone for five to fifteen minutes (or longer if you are more experienced), and adopt a comfortable seated position.

2. Begin by taking several deep, cleansing breaths, breathing in through your nose and out through your mouth. During this initial sequence, make sure you are inhaling fully into the base of your lungs so that your abdomen expands with each in-breath like a pregnant woman's belly; likewise, exhale completely, squeezing the diaphragm to push all the air, and carbon dioxide (waste), out. Try to

think of the lungs as a sponge. You need to really squeeze them to clear them out.

3. Next, as you continue to breathe deeply, with each out-breath, feel your muscles begin to relax from head to toe, focusing on one body part at a time: head, face (especially your jaw and brow), neck, and shoulders; arms, hands, and fingers; torso and hips; then your legs, feet, and toes. Allow any stored tension to drain away; then take a moment to survey your body and try to relax any areas that are still holding tension. When you start to sense the beginnings of relaxation, let your breathing return to normal. This whole relaxation sequence should take no more than about two minutes.

4. Now, begin counting your inhalations and exhalations silently to yourself. For instance, on your next in-breath, think "*one*." And then as you exhale, think "*two*." Inhale, "*three*." Exhale, "*four*."

5. Continue counting your breaths in this manner without allowing other thoughts to distract you from this simple practice. When you reach "*ten*," start over from "*one*." Also, whenever you realize that you have stopped counting and started thinking, gently but firmly return to the practice of counting your breaths, beginning from "*one*."

This is the entire practice, which should be continued throughout the duration of the meditation period. Set a timer, watch, or alarm to keep track of the time, or just open your eyes briefly to check the time. When you are finished, open your eyes and take a moment or two to readjust to the outside world, allowing the lingering sense of peace to stay with you. An important goal of meditation is to learn how to transfer the peace of your meditative practice to real-world life and its stresses.

Day 2

Today we are going to once again practice the same exercise that was introduced yesterday, zazen. Read through yesterday's instructions once more, and practice as directed. As you do so, keep in mind that the act of returning your mind to the meditation whenever you realize you've drifted into ordinary thinking patterns is an essential part of the exercise. This meditation has two parts. It is not only counting the breaths but also *returning* to counting the breaths when your mind drifts. In fact, this important second element is what especially helps develop your ability to focus. Each time you return your mind to the practice of counting your breaths, you strengthen your ability to concentrate. It's natural for the mind to wander during meditation. This can be frustrating for beginners, but don't let it bother you. Try to think of it as being like physical exercise. By focusing, losing focus, and then refocusing, you will be strengthening your mind in the same way a bodybuilder lifts and lowers weights to build muscle. It isn't a static exercise, but rather a specific, coordinated movement designed to contract and relax the muscle.

Doing this exercise will help you focus not only during meditation but also in your day-to-day life. Many people who practice meditation regularly discover that they become better able to function in the real world. You may observe other positive effects as well, such as more raw energy and increased levels of creativity.

Day 3

Today's meditations, which once again should be undertaken in the morning and evening if possible, will be very similar to those on Days 1 and 2, except that now we are going to add a key word to the mix instead of using only numbers. Counting the breaths is a simple practice that is easy to understand, and so it makes a good place to begin. Numbers are neutral, however, and so their use is more limited than words, which are known as mantras when used during meditation. While some traditions prefer the use of neutral symbols, in my experience mantras can help infuse meditative practice with a sense of meaning. Chosen with care, the right word or combination of words can encourage peace and quietness, and it can deepen your practice.

Before you begin, repeat steps 1 through 3 from Day 1. That is, find a relatively quiet place, sit comfortably, do some deep breathing, and get relaxed. None of this needs to be perfect. You may not be able to find an absolutely quiet spot, and you may not be entirely comfortable sitting still. The point of meditation is not to find perfect peace outside yourself but to cultivate a place of internal peace. Once you begin developing a space of peace within, you will be able to look outward upon chaotic situations and remain tranquil. Okay, relatively tranquil. But you're moving in the right direction! During your practice periods, just do your best to get situated and to sense the beginnings of relaxation.

When you are ready, begin counting your breaths as you did yesterday, except that now you are going to count only your inhalations. On your exhalations, instead of counting, think silently to yourself the word "*peace*." For example, as you inhale, think "*one*"; as you exhale, think "*peace*." Inhale, think "*two*"; exhale, think "*peace*."

Once again, continue counting to "*ten*" and then start over from "*one*." You should also return to "*one*" every time you realize you have stopped counting and started thinking.

Day 4

Twice today, repeat yesterday's meditation. This time, however, try focusing on the *feeling* that the word *peace* instills, allowing your body and mind to relax just a little more with each repetition of the mantra. To reiterate an earlier point, the basic meditative practice — which in this case is counting your inhalations and repeating the mantra "*peace*" during your exhalations — is only a surface goal. The real objective is to *experience* the feeling of peace that radiates from your core self, which has nothing at all to do with your ability to count. So, as you exhale and think "*peace*," try to sense that deeper place of peace within you, beyond the practice of counting the breaths.

Day 5

As already noted, the particular focus during meditation can take many forms: words, images, numbers, colors. Each technique may produce a slightly different experience, but this is true only at the shallowest levels of meditation. During deep meditation, the experiences go well beyond the forms of practice and merge into a common experience of profound inner stillness — and, ultimately, total identification with the core self and Source.

Don't get caught up in the forms of meditation. Their primary purpose is to help you achieve a state of inner peace and stillness so that you will be able to reconnect with your core, which exists deep within you in a perpetual state of peace and stillness. You need to begin matching your core's natural state in order to identify with it. The more peaceful, still, and quiet your thoughts become, the closer you get to reconnecting with your core self. Let these techniques be nothing more than a vehicle for achieving peace and stillness. As you work through each day's suggestions during the initial thirty days, pay attention to which techniques work best for you in terms of eliciting a feeling of peace.

In this spirit, for today's exercises try listening to the silent, still spaces between your thoughts. There is a stillness beyond the incessant noise of the ego-mind, a deep and powerful silence that can be intuited as your thoughts grow increasingly quiet. Let today's mantra bring your thoughts to peace, and attempt to listen with intent to the silent spaces between them. During this attempt, it is helpful to understand that we tend to think in words and sentences. Our thoughts may seem to run on and on endlessly, but sentences naturally have pauses — and so do your thoughts. Become mindful of those small breaks that appear between your thoughts. If you find it helpful, you might begin placing a mental period at the end of each sentence that passes through your mind and then focusing on those periods. Ask yourself, "What exists in the spaces between my thoughts?" The answer to this question will come to you not in words but as a feeling.

Fittingly, today's mantra is

Peace.

Repeat the word "*peace*" each time you exhale, and simultaneously allow yourself to settle more and more deeply into the feeling of inner peace and deep relaxation. Don't worry about counting your breaths. Just focus on deep relaxation.

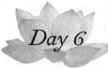

Day 6

The one-word mantra *"peace"* is short, simple, and effective. Some mantras, however, are composed of full sentences or even brief passages. Today we will use a longer mantra that focuses on helping you sense the connection between your mind and body. Often we regard these two elements of our lives as separate, but mind and body are intertwined in a fundamental and intimate dance. Today's exercise is designed to help you begin to sense this connection.

Repeat the following mantra throughout your meditation, letting the words infuse both your mind and your body with a deep and growing sense of peace and wellness, and of the connection between your mind and body. Try to feel as if with each inhalation a great sense of peace is entering your mind and soothing your thoughts, undoing any stress, anxiety, and accumulated feelings of anger. As you exhale, imagine that this sense of peace is flowing from your mind directly into your body, bringing a sense of wellness and relaxation to it, covering your skin, flowing from your head to your fingertips and all the way down to your toes, filling your lungs as you inhale and exhale, circulating through your veins, and even feeding directly into your internal organs. Imagine this sense of peace as a living, vital force that is working in both body and mind to bring healing.

As you inhale, think *"peace and stillness,"* and as you exhale, think *"mind and body."*

Repeat this mantra over and over in sync with your respiratory cycle, trying to stay focused on it and the feeling of peace, and remember to return your attention back to the practice whenever you drift into ordinary thinking.

Day 7

Today's practice is similar to yesterday's, only in abbreviated form. You can shorten or lengthen most basic mantras to suit your own preferences. Ideally, the mantra should have a nice rhythm to it, so that the flow is steady and mildly hypnotic. I like to think of a good mantra as a mental magnet designed to draw your consciousness inward toward a one-pointed focus on the present.

Like all the mantras we have been using, today's is designed to help you release negative feelings. Tapping into the peace of meditation is natural when you free yourself from tumultuous thoughts. In fact, it happens automatically, because peace is the underlying nature of life. All you need to do is learn to relax, let go of conflict thoughts, and sink into peace. This is what can make meditation so easy and natural.

As you inhale, think *"peace,"* and as you exhale, think *"still."* Inhale, *"peace,"* exhale, *"still,"* and so on.

As before, try focusing on the *feeling* of peace, and let it grow with each repetition of the mantra, as if the mantra itself were a living, magnetic energy attracting your mind toward its natural underlying state of quietness.

Day 8

There comes a time when every meditation student wonders if he or she is meditating "correctly." We all go through this stage, typically early on. Thoughts can bombard you with such tenacity that sometimes it may seem as if you are getting nowhere — and the practice is so very different from any other activity that it can at times feel a little pointless. Perhaps you've already experienced some of this. While instant, or at least rapid, success is possible in meditation, it's more common to feel some level of frustration at the beginning.

If this has been the case for you, take heart. As long as you are making the effort to practice daily, you'll advance. Whether or not you are aware of it, there is a great Power within you, and every time you sit down to practice, that Power reaches out and tries to connect with you. Because of this, even the bumbling attempts of the most inexperienced student are always successful to some degree. You cannot sit down to meditate and fail entirely. It simply is not possible. There will be times, no doubt about it, when you will feel frustrated, as if you are getting nowhere, and so far removed from peace that you cannot fathom how you have accomplished anything. Yet, however much you think this to be the case, you are wrong. The tiniest shift toward core self *always* produces results. In fact, it is often the times when we are struggling the most that our greatest successes are achieved. For when you are succeeding at meditation, your ego will feel threatened. Because of this, as you approach your greatest breakthroughs, you may judge your practice as being at its lowest point.

So don't worry if you haven't instantly taken to the practice or you feel a little confused as to what you are *supposed* to be feeling during meditation. Things will get clearer as you go along. In the meantime, trust sustained daily practice to see you through. And as I said earlier, if it feels like a chore right now, that's okay. Meditation is one of the best things you can do for your health, and the benefits certainly outweigh the small investment of time it requires. Even if you are uncertain or confused, you will still attain the physical and emotional benefits of meditation as long as you are taking the time to practice. It can be hard to accept, but intellectual understanding is not essential to meditation. We Westerners in particular hate to hear that, but it is still the truth. You don't have to understand meditation any more than you have to understand what makes the sun shine in order to appreciate a beautiful day at the beach.

Today's mantra is just a little different from those we have already tried. It includes an additional part, so that it will be done in four parts spread out over two complete inhalation/exhalation cycles. When you are ready and relaxed, on your next in-breath, think "*Breathing in, my body fills with light.*" As you exhale, think "*Breathing out, I find myself at peace.*" Then, on the next in-breath, think "*Breathing in, my mind fills with joy,*" and finally, "*Breathing out, I realize that I am the joy.*"

Day 9

Contrast is a powerful teacher. A mind at peace is quiet and still, whereas conflict thoughts are noisy, brash, and grating. This may seem obvious, but what is less clear is that we have a choice in the types of thoughts we allow to occupy our minds. Your mind, your thoughts, and your feelings should be your most treasured assets, along with the people you love. Your thoughts have a mighty, incalculable effect on the events you experience. You wouldn't allow someone to live in your home if you knew the person was going to be highly disruptive and destructive to your property, would you? Probably not. By allowing thoughts of hostility, sadness, guilt, fear, and the many other forms that darkness may take to occupy a place in your mind, you are actively inviting a most unwelcome guest into your home of homes. Your mind is a sacred space, and if you have not already adopted this attitude, I invite you to do so now.

By learning how to meditate, you are also learning the art of *conscious living*. Conscious living means that you do not allow your life to just happen. Instead, you actively and intentionally manage your life. Think of it this way — you wouldn't get into your car, fire up the engine, and kick it into gear without being prepared to take the wheel. Your car, at least for the time being, is not going to steer itself. So why would you live your life aimlessly, merely reacting to the events that were thrust upon you instead of taking the lead to shape those events?

One way to begin living consciously is to meditate every morning. By doing so, you are, in a sense, declaring your intention to live consciously. You can also use your morning meditation to clarify the type of day you would like to have. Spend just a minute or two of your morning meditation to tell yourself what types of things you want to experience in the day to come, the type of life you want to live, how you want others to view you, and the types of interactions you would like to have with the people in your life. For instance, do you want a day of peace and quiet reflection filled with powerful life lessons, inspiration, and genuine connection with other people? A day during which you feel loved, respected, and valuable? A day of sharing; of open, fearless giving and receiving; of intimate communication and forward progress? If so, make sure you set this intention into motion first thing in the morning.

Today's thought of peace, which is once again a four-part meditation to be synced with your breath, is

Breathing in, I am filled with tranquillity;
breathing out, my mind is very quiet; breathing in,
stillness surrounds me; breathing out, I am stillness.

Day 10

Now that you've had some experience with meditation, let's go back to an earlier lesson. For today's practice, once again try counting your breaths, both the inhalations and exhalations, as you did on Day 1, except do not stop at "*ten*." Instead, just continue counting as high as possible before you lose concentration. When this happens, you may begin again from "*one*." Compare your experience now with that which you had when you first tried it. Is it easier or more difficult? You might even think of this practice as a mental game: How high are you able to count before you have to start over from "*one*"?

Overcoming Obstacles

F ear actively blocks your awareness of core self. Other negative emotional states, especially guilt and anger, which are both closely related to fear, have the same effect.

One night, an old Cherokee man was sitting around a campfire, teaching his grandchildren about the lessons he had learned in life and the lessons they would also need to learn. "There is a great battle being waged within me. It is a fight between two wolves," he said, speaking gently but with intensity. "One wolf represents anger, envy, sorrow, regret, greed, arrogance, self-pity, guilt, resentment, inferiority, lies, false pride, competition, superiority, and ego." The grandfather was quiet for a minute, allowing the children to process this, before he continued. "And the other wolf stands for joy, peace, love, hope, serenity, humility, kindness, benevolence, empathy, generosity, truth, compassion, and faith." Then he looked at each of the children directly, one by one, meeting and holding their eyes. "This same struggle is raging inside each of you too, and in everyone."

At this point the grandfather fell into a deep silence, his eyes on the fire as sparks drifted into the air and faded into the star-filled sky. Some time passed, and still none of the children disturbed their grandfather, for they knew he had the ability to turn inward and see beyond the veil of the world, into other worlds. The silence stretched out like a tightening band until one of the boys — the youngest of them, who in his innocence had not developed the patience of the others — could stand it no longer. "But Grandfather," the boy blurted out at last, "which wolf will win? Which one?"

The grandfather shifted his gaze, looked gently upon the boy, and shrugged. "Whichever one you feed," he said.

This Native American legend reflects a truth that many have realized: there are indeed two forces within us, representing directly opposite viewpoints. Even today, this is reflected in our own storytelling. For instance, as a kid who grew up in the seventies and eighties, I fell in love with the *Star Wars* movies, like so many of my generation. Not only did these films launch my imagination into a galaxy far, far away, but they also echoed spiritual truths that are a part of the collective unconscious of the human race. In the films, an epic battle is, of course, being waged between good and evil powers, and the "Force" — the engine behind the story — is a great invisible power that runs like a river throughout the universe, throughout life. Both the heroes and the villains of the pictures are those who have learned how to tap into the Force and use its power for either darkness or light, evil or good. More recently, the *Harry Potter* series captured the imaginations of millions of readers and moviegoers, old and young, by presenting similar themes.

When you are watching films and reading books like these, what you are seeing on the screen or page is more than just a projection of light passed through film or words on a page. It is a projection from our inner, collective unconscious. These stories depict a truth about the universe that we intuit on a deep and basic level. A struggle between the forces of good and evil has been going on in our world at least since early recorded history. When you look more closely at the nature of conflict, however, you will begin to realize that the wars being fought outside of us find their origin inside of us. Just as the Native American story above relates, a civil war *is* being fought within each one of us. It isn't just countries that fight each other. We are fighting against ourselves. The outward manifestations of this war — whether they come out as physical violence or emotional violence between either nations or individuals — are the physical expressions of an ancient inner disease. We don't really need to solve the conflicts between nations, then, but only the conflict that exists within each of us as individuals.

Meditation is a powerful spotlight into the soul. It is a practice by which we shut down these outward projections and flip the light of our consciousness around to shine inward and illuminate our inner psychological and spiritual landscape. When we do this, we gradually begin to perceive the two wolves at war within us, and through this clear recognition we can at last begin consciously choosing which wolf we will "feed." Until we recognize that the wars we experience in the external world are caused by our internal state, we will never be able to come to peace on either a personal or a global level.

So how do you feed your wolf of choice? Very simply. You love it. You invest in it. You think about it every day and invite it to take an active part in every decision you make. When you look upon another person, you turn to the Wolf of Light and ask, "How shall I view this person?" When you look upon the events of your life, you ask the wolf, "How shall I view this happening?" And when you make a decision, you say, "Which path is the path of light?" Basically, you feed the Wolf of Light through your day-to-day choices, your thoughts, and your love.

I said before that we may experience tremendous resistance to meditation, and there is a reason for this. By feeding the Wolf of Light, we are simultaneously starving the Wolf of Darkness. Put another way, by investing in light, you are eliminating darkness in the same way that turning on a light at night automatically causes darkness to vanish. At first this can feel like a loss, as if you are losing some major aspect of yourself. The sudden appearance of light can be a shock. Even on a physical level, a light turned on in a darkened room hurts our eyes until they adjust. But imagine what the experience would be like for people who had spent their *entire lives* locked away in a prison of darkness and knew of nothing else. They might well be terrified.

In our world, this is much like the position we find ourselves in. It takes a while to adjust to the light of deep meditation — and to learn that this new awareness is perfectly safe and, what's more, that it brings real joy.

To learn how to meditate, then, you are going to have to deal with this resistance within yourself — your own battle between good and evil. For meditation is very much a shift into light, because it is a shift into understanding our deepest nature. In our world, we see only with our eyes, which are designed to register the outside world. In a sense, this keeps us blind to our inner self, just as if we were living in a darkened prison. Yet darkness and light cannot exist within you at the same time. You experience one or the other all the time, *but only one in any given instant.* So, as you advance toward the light of understanding that meditation yields, the Wolf of Darkness feels threatened. It will seek to persuade you to stop meditating or will interfere with your practicing in any way you allow it to.

During the practice of meditation, the most common forms of this resistance are restlessness, an inability to focus, physical discomfort, anxiety, hyperactive thoughts (also known as *monkey mind*), drowsiness (which is monkey mind's opposite), and the many related symptoms. Virtually any thought or feeling that will keep you from going too deeply within, toward core self, will suffice. The Wolf of Darkness is not at all concerned with the forms of resistance, so long as they work. This resistance is insidious and highly active, and it will seek to thwart your efforts in any way that gets you to respond, although it has absolutely no power to stop you. The efforts of the Wolf of Darkness rely on smoke and mirrors, but nothing more substantial.

Subtler forms of resistance, besides the obvious physical and psychological symptoms, may occur during the act of meditation.

These may seek to persuade you to stop meditating *permanently*. At some point, for instance, the Wolf of Darkness might whisper to you things like "Meditation is just *not for you*; you are *too busy*; you can't learn it because your mind is *too restless*." Or perhaps it might take a different approach: "It's not doing anything. You are wasting your time." Or maybe, just a bit further down the road, it might even try to convince you that you have advanced "beyond the need for structured practice." I have seen many students fall prey to this tired old line. The point is, there are many such sweet nothings, each one as senseless as the rest.

Simply put, the Wolf of Darkness may apply any tactic to get you to stop meditating. This force is persistent, and it can be quite ingenious. Here I have pointed out only a few of the more common versions its story can take. Because the Wolf of Darkness is not an outside force but a product of your own mind, it is as intelligent and logical as you are. You can't underestimate it. If you hope to develop a long-term meditative practice, you will need to become aware of its tricks and learn to ignore them. Without your allegiance, all forms of resistance will come and go without effect.

Whenever you are struggling with your meditative practice, recognize that you are merely experiencing the ancient battle between light and darkness, which has always been around, and become determined to press through it. Gradually, very gently, this struggle will subside as long as you remain determined and set. Become a stubborn meditator, and the Wolf of Darkness will have no power over you. Second, work daily on feeding the Wolf of Light. Actively seek out exercises that help you to embrace peaceful, loving thoughts and attitudes. Allow thoughts of forgiveness to replace thoughts of condemnation. Allow thoughts of trust to replace thoughts of fear. Choose thoughts of innocence instead of thoughts of guilt. Become an active participant in this transition. Meditate every day, and center your awareness with core self. This will help you to balance your emotions so that you are not swinging wildly between states of pain and states of peace. Most important, devote yourself to living a conscious life that is absolutely dedicated to growing into the most radiant, peaceful person you are capable of being. Of course, you will fail many times, but "failure" per se is always temporary. In fact, I prefer the notion that there is no such thing as failure, only lessons to learn along the way to success.

The Three Tales of the Wolf of Darkness

As your meditative practice progresses, it is important to learn to recognize the forms that resistance may take. The truth is, the obstacles only *seem* to be many. They are all based on three primary stages of development. Don't let the forms deceive you. Just as the Wolf of Darkness isn't concerned with which form of his story you buy into, you shouldn't be concerned with form, either.

Body Identification

The first story the Wolf of Darkness will tell you is that you are your body and nothing more. This is the most basic form of resistance to meditation, and it includes any thought or experience that increases the feeling of body identification. During meditation, you are switching your focus from body identification toward Spirit identification. It is helpful, therefore, to begin to view your body as only a small part of what you really are, and not your core self at all. The body is best thought of as a temporary extension of the core self, used during our time on earth as a learning tool. While you are focused on the body's senses, needs, and experiences, you will remain tied to it and will believe that it *is you*. This inevitably makes meditation seem fearful, even though it is anything but, because the practice reminds you quite directly that there is more to you than this temporary mass of flesh, blood, and bones. Thus meditation challenges the Wolf of Darkness's first line of defense.

It isn't surprising that the forms of resistance related to the need to preserve body identification typically involve those that increase your awareness of the body and its needs. There is no subtlety about this process. These may include aches and pains, itches, shortness of breath, illness, and various other physical phenomena. Resistance may also come in the form of thoughts about the body and its needs and wants, which might include a rash of bodily fears and desires. Whatever the forms, learn to recognize them as nothing more than the Wolf of Darkness's story that you are your body and your body is you.

In response, I suggest that you embrace the following notion and learn to hold it dear to your heart: *I am not my body. I am Spirit.* Memorize these two short, simple sentences, and think of them every day. They speak a hidden truth about you that will one day bring you great joy and release. The trick is learning that these words are true, which you can do only through experience. By turning inward in meditation, you are seeking exactly this.

It is also important to note here that your attempts to reach inward and go beyond the body do not endanger it. On the contrary, as we will explore more deeply later, opening to meditation naturally heals the body. So have no fear about releasing your identification with the body. Go as deeply as you can in meditation, and the body will only be strengthened by your experiences. It will still be around when you return.

Thought Identification

As you release your identification with the body, the next story the Wolf of Darkness will tell you is that if you are not your body, then you must be your individual thoughts and personality. We are always seeking a sense of self, and since the existence of the Wolf of Darkness (the ego) is based on individual personality, it must remain broken off from the greater body of Life. This must be true, because as you approach your core self, which is a direct, original reflection of Source, your sense of individuality gradually dissolves. The waterfall of thoughts in the ego-mind, then, becomes our second hang-up on the journey inward.

This presents a double-edged problem. First, as mentioned

everyday meditation

before, our thoughts run nonstop, like a cascading veil that hides the world beyond them. There appears to be no way through. Second, we are very much inclined to latch on to our thoughts anyway, for what would we "be" without all our individual thoughts? This question must arise, and it instantly increases the threat level in the ego.

The way past this avalanche of thought is not through force of any kind. Releasing this obstacle and finding your way clear instead involves reprogramming the content of the waterfall itself. You will observe, as you sit in meditation watching the stunning force of your own personal waterfall of thoughts, that quite a lot, if not most, of these thoughts are composed of negative emotions. Fear, anger, and guilt thoughts are among the most common, though they often masquerade as more moderate — or even kindly — thoughts. These negative emotions are so fearful that you will naturally be repulsed by them, and so you will not seek to challenge them and go beyond them. This is a natural enough reaction, and it is exactly why reprogramming the thought system of the mind is essential. We will discuss techniques for doing this later. For now, it is important to note the phenomenon and to become aware of it — and, most important, to begin drawing a distinction between you and your thoughts. They are not the same, just as you are not your body. Ultimately, you will find the greatest success in meditation by letting your negative thoughts be transformed into thoughts based on forgiveness, compassion, and unconditional love. Such positive thoughts lack the fearful nature of fear-based ones, thus reducing resistance to connecting with your core self. They are still just thoughts, but the switch is an essential step in the process of going beyond all individual thoughts.

Fear of Loss of Identity

After you have realized that you are not your body and you are not your thoughts, what does the Wolf of Darkness tell you? Here is the real obstacle behind the others, which were in place only to keep this one, ultimate obstacle hidden. The loss of our sense of self is the ultimate human fear, and therefore the ultimate threat from this viewpoint must be Spirit, which in its vastness encompasses the whole body of life — everyone and all creatures, all true thought, every galaxy and universe, and all levels of life, both corporeal and noncorporeal. Think of the implications! Spirit is the exact opposite of the state of separation. It is a state in which life is experienced directly as a perfect, eternal union and continuous expansion. Therefore, no sense of individual self can be long maintained within it. In the deepest meditative states, the little ego-self is temporarily swept away and grows indistinguishable within Spirit, just as it would be impossible to distinguish a single drop of water in an ocean.

This may sound frightening, but it is actually anything but. In any case, the experience is temporary, and in fact it purifies you each time you let go and immerse yourself in the spiritual world. This always empowers you and never takes away. You never lose anything in this exchange.

The way to undo this fear of loss of self is through experience. Until you realize that relinquishing identification with your individual self is not a loss — which you can do only through your own experience — you will be apt to look upon the ocean of life as an incomprehensible, alien expanse. You will be afraid that if you were to completely let go, your little self would be swept away forever. This is the biggest fear, the greatest obstacle, that needs to be undone if you are to experience the release of deepest meditation. Whatever else your problems with meditation seem to be, this is the only one you need concern yourself with. Seek only to release this fear and develop trust, and you will advance far into your meditative experience.

Day 11

So far, we have tried two related forms of meditation, zazen and silent mantra (some mantras are recited aloud). The next series of meditations will take our practicing in a different direction, adding a new dimension to it. Instead of using words as a central focus, we are now going to use images. The fundamental principle of visualization is the same as that of mantra — keep your mind focused on your practice to the exclusion of interrupting thoughts. Also, the meditations will still have two parts to them: the attempt to maintain your concentration on the specific exercise, and the effort you make to return to your practice when your mind drifts into unrelated thoughts. As before, both aspects should be considered equally valuable.

For today's meditations, begin as usual by closing your eyes and getting comfortable and relaxed. Next, imagine yourself meditating before a great ocean, the water gently lapping on the shore, the sun warm but not hot, the day quiet. You are at peace here, safe and perfectly still, sensing your oneness with the expanse of water that stretches out toward infinity. During this exercise, try to reach out and sense your unity, not only with the ocean but with all the life it contains and supports as well. You are also at one with the sky and with the birds that wheel and dive above the waters, with the sound of the waves lapping on the shore, and with everything and everyone that happens to cross your mind during this meditation. Notice how there is a natural rhythm to the ocean. The waves roll onto the shore in sets. The tides rise and fall, just like your breath. Try to see how you too are a part of the natural cycles of life.

Meditate on this sense of unity with the ocean and sky

throughout your practicing, and, as usual, whenever you realize that you have lost focus, return your attention once again to the image of sitting before the sea, relaxing in peace and oneness. The image itself is nothing. It is the peace the image brings to mind that will help you to make the deeper connection with core self.

Day 12

Today, focus once again on the same image you used yesterday. This time, however, you are going to add one more element to the visualization: Whenever you realize that you are thinking and have allowed your mind to stray from your practice, instead of merely returning your attention to the image of the ocean, take a moment to identify the fact that you have allowed your mind to drift into ordinary thinking. Do this by imagining the word *"thinking"* being drawn in the wet sand at your feet. You may imagine yourself writing the word with your finger, or you can just imagine it appearing as if by magic. Either way, just take a few seconds to see the word written in the sand as clearly as you can. Then imagine a little wave sweeping in and washing it away, and pull your attention back toward the open sea as the waters retreat.

One of the challenges you'll encounter during meditation is catching your mind when it has wandered. This is not always easy to do. Today's exercise is intended to improve your ability to notice when this happens, as well as to give you an additional nudge back into the visualization by providing an intermediary visual exercise.

Day 13

Now let us switch venues from the ocean to a wooded river-bank. This time, watch quietly as the water flows downstream past you. Once again, imagine a peaceful, safe setting, sheltered by trees and warmed by a mild sun. The sound of the river and its passage will provide the focus for your meditation. Allow your whole consciousness to become absorbed in the river's powerful flow, which also makes a good analogy for life. The river is steady and yet always changing, like time and space. It is a little body of water compared with the sea, but it flows on and out of sight, eventually joining the sea, just as we join a greater body of life, our own Source, somewhere beyond our everyday awareness. Also, the river's flow may wax and wane, and the river itself may either dry up or swell and overrun its banks, but in either case, these are only illusions of change. The water is the substance behind the river's life, and this is never truly lost. Even when the river appears to be dried up, the water has only temporarily retreated into hiding. It has seeped into the soil, nurturing the trees, animals, and plants; or it has been taken up into the sky, where it waits to fall back to the earth again as rain and snow. And so it is with our core self, which is never lost and never truly changes. Even when we cannot see it, it is still a part of us. We just need to learn how to shift our focus to become aware of it.

Day 14

Now try taking the riverside meditation one step further, just as you did with the ocean meditation. This time, as you meditate on the river's passage, when you catch yourself thinking, imagine your thoughts as leaves appearing in an eddy of swirling water near the river's bank. There they are trapped temporarily, dancing and twirling in the water, until at last the river's pull wins out and sends them racing downstream and out of sight. Let them go, along with the thoughts they represent in your mind. This is exactly how you should deal with thoughts during meditation — and during everyday life, for that matter: as temporary, flowing energy that can be used at times, but that you have no need to cling to. As you learn how to free your thinking in this way, you will begin to sense a newborn emotional stability. Constant emotional involvement with our passing thoughts causes us an incredible amount of stress and anxiety, whereas learning to let our thoughts flow smoothly past without attachment is the heart of liberation.

Day 15

The purpose of visualization is not only to provide a place to keep your mind anchored, thus bringing a sense of order to its disorderly state, but also, most important, to inspire a sense of peace through which it becomes easier to open to the meditative experience. We have made this point before. Mantras do this same thing, only with words — either through their literal meaning, such as "*peace*," or their sound and rhythm, such as the beautiful Buddhist chant "*Gate, gate, paragate, parasamgate, bodhi svaha.*" They are intended, at least in part, to soothe the mind. I like to think of visualization images as *picture mantras*, since their purpose is much the same. Just like mantras, the images used during visualization are merely tools that assist you in reaching a deep enough state of peace that you are able to realign with core self. Since core self exists in a deep, immutable state of peace, the quieter and more peaceful you are, the closer you come to merging your full awareness with it. This point is so important to understand that it will be repeated many times, in different ways, throughout this training program.

Today we are going to try a slightly different style of visualization, one that steps away from explicit pictures of external settings, such as the river and ocean, and turns in the natural direction of meditation — back toward us, inward.

Picture yourself meditating in an empty, golden-hued room that is filled with nothing but the softest of natural light. Here there is nothing for you to focus on except your own body, your mind, and this room with its warm light. As you look closer, notice that the room is not composed of hard and fixed walls at all but is *made of* the light that fills it and surrounds you. It is literally a room of light.

Next, meditate on the thought that you and this room are one, and that your own body is not composed of flesh at all but is also made of this same light. Furthermore, this light does not end at the room's walls. It stretches forever — both outward, around the world and into outer space, and inward, through you and into inner space. Let this image be a bridge to help you to begin to experience what it must mean to be a being of light, with no boundaries, no walls, and no limits.

Day 16

Meditation is not a matter of concentration; it is a matter of peace. When you are at peace, meditation is easy, but when you are in conflict, your meditations will hit a wall. By now, you surely have started to notice that peace is a major theme of this book. Some traditional meditation teachings emphasize concentration exercises, but if you choose only to develop your ability to focus without regard to the cultivation of quietness of thought, your progress will be severely hampered. An infinitely more effective approach to learning meditation is to focus specifically on the development of peace, because to meditate deeply, you need not learn how to *focus* per se. You only need to learn the gentle art of unconditional love, simple kindness, and compassionate action and thought.

This is true because meditation *is* a movement into deepening states of peace. In fact, you could rightly describe the practice as the effort to release all conflict and immerse yourself directly in peace. This is why when you are upset — regardless of the form or degree of the upset — meditation can seem impossible. In such a state, your thoughts go wild as you try to sink into the quiet sphere of meditation, rebelling against your efforts as if they had a will of their own. During such times, it may seem as if the attempt to meditate is causing you to feel even more upset. This is only a perception, of course, not a fact.

By regularly attempting to bring your mind to a state of peace, you are confronting all the negative things that have built up over a lifetime of hurts, fears, and regrets. It is all this internal garbage that we need to work through and get rid of. These wounds — whether they are self-inflicted or appear to have been caused by other people or external circumstances — and the guilt, fear, and anger they arouse, are the real obstacle to stillness, not a lack of concentration. Another important point here is that meditation does not *cause* these emotions, which are already present and silently poison our lives and relationships every day. Meditation merely makes you more aware of them. It brings them out into the open so that you can heal them. While they remain buried in unconsciousness, they cause all types of problems, from anxiety and depression to heart disease and divorce. Left unhealed, these dark wounds — even when you are not aware of them — bleed into your daily life all the time, and they cannot help but wreak havoc. Cleansing your life of this stuff is the real work not only of meditative practice but also of any genuine healing. It may be the most important project of your life, and very few people choose to undertake it. If they did, this world would be a vastly different place.

Be thankful that you have the opportunity today to work through a little more of your own internal garbage and to free yourself of it. As you push further toward your core self with each meditation you undertake daily, you challenge more of your own unhealed wounds, and where the peace of your meditation meets these old wounds, you heal. Think of these exercises as medicine for your psyche, applied deep down near the site of the problem.

Begin your meditations today as usual, and then try to imagine a light building within your center — a subtle golden glow much like the light you focused on yesterday. Imagine it first in your chest region, and then let this light gradually expand until it fills your entire body: down the length of your arms to the tips of your fingers, into your legs and feet, and up and over your head, wrapping you in a cocoon of light. It is warm and gentle, and it brings you a renewed sense of balance and vitality.

Spend the remainder of the meditation focusing on this light and your unity with it, recalling your mind to the image and associated feelings whenever you feel your attention wander. Once again, try to gain a sense that you are composed not of flesh and blood, but of light that fills the universe.

Day 17

Sometimes people feel guilty about things they are doing exclusively for themselves. This happens often when it comes to meditation. Because you are setting aside time away from friends, family, school, work, and just about everything else the world deems important, you may feel a little guilty.

Don't allow yourself to feel guilty about meditating. By taking the time to meditate, you are doing a favor not only for yourself but for everybody else in your life as well. If you think there is any aspect of your life that won't benefit from your practice, you are listening to your ego. Everyone you know will benefit from your meditative practice in one way or another, because when you improve yourself, your relationships will improve automatically. This is a given. You will feel less conflict and more peace — and it should be no surprise that this will be reflected in how you deal with others, especially during moments of stress and conflict. So your meditative practice is also good for your kids, your spouse, your friends, your coworkers, your boss, and everyone else in your life. It isn't only for self-healing.

You will probably also discover that, over time, you will become a more creative and intuitive person who is increasingly productive. By doing the inner work to fix your own life, you are also going to affect all the circumstances of your outer life. Gradually, you'll begin to think more clearly; you'll feel healthier; you'll need fewer medications and doctor visits (which equates to more money); you'll be more in touch with your true emotions and feel less need to engage in melodrama — and all this is just the tip of the iceberg.

So give yourself permission up front to take as much time as you like for meditation and to feel 100 percent guilt free about doing so. By building that healthier you, you are building health-ier relationships and life circumstances as peace expands through you and extends to all the circumstances of your life.

Today, once again imagine a golden light glowing brightly within you, and see it slowly fill your body from head to toe. Next, imagine your closest friends and family members surround-ing you in a circle. Spend a minute or two meditating on this image, seeing it as clearly as possible. Finally, see the light begin radiating from you, gradually creating a brilliant, living mist all around. This healing light then moves to surround those you love as well and covers their skin, gradually becoming one with them too. Imagine it filling their bodies and bringing them to a state of intense inner peace, balance, and healing. Everyone this light touches finds healing in whatever form they need.

Also notice how the light unites you all — your loved ones with one another and you with them. Spend the remainder of your meditation focusing on the feeling of being united and at peace with everyone in your life through light, and bear in mind that this fantasy is only one part make-believe. There is an element of truth to it, for it reflects the unity that does connect us with one another and is the real channel of healing between us.

Day 18

Some forms of meditation use certain subtle locations of the body as their focus. These are called the *chakras*. Technically, they are not physical locations, but it is easier for most people to think of them that way. At a glance, the body appears solid, but it is much subtler than gross matter. This is why meditation students commonly report the sensation of shifting energy currents throughout their body, particularly in the beginning and intermediate stages of development. The body is actually composed of organized energy, and it isn't a stable, fixed system but rather one that is in a constant state of flux. During meditation, you become more aware of these shifts. Rest assured, these feelings will not last long.

Perhaps this all sounds rather magical to you. I once thought so myself. However, after much experience I've come to realize that there is a certain amount of truth to the whole business of the chakras. There do, in fact, seem to be naturally occurring hubs of energy within the body, which I like to think of as energy vortices; and when you focus on them, you can produce powerful meditative experiences.

Besides shifting energy, during meditation you may have other physical sensations, such as numbness or a feeling of sudden detachment from your body. This is perfectly normal. Learn to relax and don't be afraid of these experiences. You are merely passing beyond body identification.

The chakras can be thought of as a series of interconnected pools of energy that exist at key locations in the subtler energy field of the body. You might try thinking of them as subtle organs made of pure energy, linked by a chain of flowing energy. It isn't the purpose of this book to provide detailed instruction regarding the chakras; however, three key locations are often used during meditation. These are the heart chakra, the third eye chakra, and the crown chakra. Today's practice will focus on the heart chakra. The other two will be discussed over the next two days.

- The *heart chakra* is the center of emotional well-being and represents our capacity to give and receive love.

You can easily meditate on the heart chakra by focusing your attention on the center of your chest. The idea is to keep your awareness attuned to this area and to try to get a feeling for the energy of this sacred center. Once you have focused your attention midchest, silently tell your heart,

I love.

Repeat this mantra with each exhalation, trying to sense the energy in your heart as a green-hued light that radiates from your chest throughout your being. Most important, try to sense the intangible feeling of love, which can be felt most strongly in this region. Some people like to visualize the heart chakra as a glowing green emerald (green being the color most closely associated with this chakra), feeding its energy of love up and down the chakra pathway (roughly paralleling the spinal column) to the other chakras. Use this meditation to tap into the sense of being loved and cared for by the universe, learning to let love flow freely throughout your being.

Also note that with today's meditation, you are learning how to combine three forms of meditation at once. Chakra, mantra, and visualization meditation all come into play here.

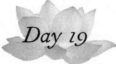

Day 19

- The *third eye chakra* is situated approximately at the point between the eyebrows. Although many believe it correlates best to intuition, its most helpful function is spiritual insight. The third eye can be thought of as "the eye that looks inward," away from the physical and toward the internal, spiritual realm. Therefore, by focusing your attention on this point, you are stimulating spiritual vision. The third eye is the most commonly used of the chakras for meditative purposes, and it is well known to evoke strong experiences.

With your eyes closed, start by focusing your awareness on the point between your eyebrows. If it helps, you may gently turn your physical eyes, although they are closed, in a slightly upward direction, as if you are trying to look toward the sky. Some people also prefer to focus their attention on their forehead, giving themselves a wider target to aim for. Then, with your next exhalation, silently begin repeating the mantra

I see.

As you did yesterday, repeat today's mantra with each exhalation, making a consistent effort to keep focused on the third eye.

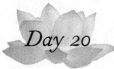

Day 20

- The *crown chakra* is thought to exist at the very top of the head. Some people believe it is the most direct link to our higher self and Source.

Keep your attention focused on the crown of your head, and think to yourself with each out-breath,

I know.

Most important, try to sense what it would feel like to exist in a state without the constant thoughts that bombard your mind. Reach out intuitively and sense yourself as pure Spirit, pure energy, pure knowing.

You may observe that by concentrating on the different chakras, you induce slightly different experiences. Note the differences and similarities, which worked best for you, and, just as important, which was most difficult.

If you like, you can combine chakra meditations with other practices like mantra, as you have tried over the last few days, or visualization, as you have also tried. Alternatively, you can make focusing on the chakra the entire practice, using no mantra or visualization. In this case, the object would be to try to tune in and align your awareness with the chakra point while quieting your mind — a bit like tuning in to a specific radio station. You adjust the dial slowly until the static clears, a process that simultaneously excludes, or tunes out, other thoughts.

The Development of Peace

Core self exists in a permanent, unalterable love-based condition; therefore, you have to be in a state of love to align with it.

Peace is taking over the world. I know it doesn't appear that way, but appearances are often deceptive. I have seen the future. I've seen it in myself and in many others as well. I know how peace feels, how it seduces you. I can look out across the world, with all its meaningless wars and moral atrocities, and there, in the midst of the chaos, I can envision the quiet, humble beginning of peace's global rule.

At some point, everyone will give in to peace. Why? Because the alternative is so exhausting and so utterly pointless that there is no alternative when you evaluate the options and look at the grand scheme. Just consider what it is we are fighting about. Most wars center around the physical, something the ego wishes to possess or defend, because it is only at this level that we can be endangered. Spirit is never in danger and never in need, and so when we are engaged with it — that is, when we realize that every one of us is a beloved aspect of One Spirit — there is no need to fight. There is no threat, and there is no lack in Spirit, and as a result there is no motivation to war. Why would we expend the energy? So, when I say I've seen the future, this is what I mean:

Our future, yours and mine and everyone's, exists within Spirit, the Origin from which we all derived and to which we will all one day return. Essentially, what's going to happen is that everyone in the world will one day simply lose the will to continue fighting and hating each other, because as we evolve as a species, we will gradually realize that there is neither need for nor reward in conflict.

When I say *everyone* will eventually give in to peace, of course I don't mean every individual who is alive today. Naturally, many of us will live out our present lifetimes in a state of conflict without ever realizing the beauty that surrounds and cares for us each day. However, societies across the world will gradually evolve toward peace, and in this way peace will spread across the globe. The only question is, how long will this evolution take? And the answer is, it shouldn't matter to you personally. You can do only your own part. You cannot change the world outside you, but you certainly *can* take charge of the one within. In fact, if you wish to be at peace, you *must* take charge of your life.

Peace is a real force. It is much more than a lack of conflict. When the desire for conflict is relinquished, peace fills the void as a living, active presence. Expressed fully, peace is the same force as Love, Spirit, Source, because true peace comes from Source. When you align yourself with peace, you are also aligning yourself with the great creative energy of Source, which underlies and expands continuously throughout the living universe. How does this alignment happen? Very simply! When you begin coming to peace with the people in your life, with yourself, and with the world, you enter a state through which you can, at last, accept your perfect unity with everyone and everything in the universe. This means you are accepting unity not with the insane behavior that occurs but rather with the core self of others, which represents their true self. Conflict and chaos always stem from ego. When you accept your unity with others, you see beyond all the madness of ego and look directly into their soul. Unity is natural when you are at peace, because you have no worries and no judgments to hold anything apart from you. That's what peace really means: no conflict on any level, either with others or within yourself. When you are at peace, you are perfectly content with your present moment, with those who share your life, and with your position in the world just as it is, right here, right now.

And you wouldn't change a thing. Think of the level of contentment such a state implies!

Peace offers you joy. When you are at peace, you smile more often. You laugh more easily. A light can be seen flitting about your eyes. You are, quite simply, happy to be right where you are, and right who you are. The state of peace brings with it a certain lightness to your step and a serenity to your face and eyes. Perhaps most important, however, is the internal experience of peace, through which you realize that your life has a purpose, one so powerful that it will one day bring unity of thought to all the nations of the world. Through its sublime beauty, which is its true power, the thought of peace will one day take over the world by taking over our hearts.

One by one, we will all give in to the healing power of peace, and one by one, the world will be transformed through us, you and me. Once experienced deeply, peace will attract you like nothing you have ever felt before, or even imagined. It is just that powerful. It will enchant you to the point where you will give up all desire to attack, just for one more taste of the release that comes from having a peaceful heart.

How is this transformation accomplished? Two ways. First, it happens when we realize that more often than not, it isn't other people's actions that harm us but our own hateful thoughts. The powerful influence of our thoughts on our feelings will be covered in a later chapter, "The Law of Reciprocity," but the important point here is that the thoughts you hold in your mind consist of pure creative energy, and they shape your entire experience of life. They are, in grand respect, the carpenters of your life. Every day, you shape your life, your experiences, and your relationships on every level through your thinking.

Of course, this does not mean that other people don't attack us on the physical and ego levels at times — but even here, we don't see how much and how often our own behavior and lack of peace encourage such attacks. We can do much to disarm other people's animosity by loosening our own investment in ego.

Second, you begin to accept peace as a lifestyle choice when you fully understand the alternative. You can be in one of only two states of mind at any given moment, *peace* or *conflict*, and one brings with it all types of blessings, while the other brings all types of hell. Ultimately, you make the switch to gentleness when you realize that it makes you happy, while its opposite brings you pain. Accepting peace is as simple as that. As was noted earlier, contrast is a mighty teacher.

Human beings have been killing each other since before recorded history, and it seems there will always be some war, somewhere. Even if we set aside the bloodshed that occurs every day of every year somewhere on the planet, peace can seem equally unfathomable closer to home. We fight with our neighbors; we fight with strangers; we fight with our coworkers, friends, mothers, brothers, and lovers. We fight with ourselves on an internal level. These attacks can include more subtle levels of assault too. Lack of peace is an *emotional state*, first and foremost. Physical violence may or may not follow the desire to attack, but the impulse always precedes physical conflict.

Besides physical aggression, we wage war with our words and passive-aggressive actions. We can even attack with our attitude, by making cruel jokes, and through well-timed, stewing silences. All of these are lesser forms of attack, but they are just as disruptive to our connection with core self and Source. Understand fully, once anger enters your mind, it is already looking for a way out — a target — *and it will find it*. Who or what that target is doesn't really matter. Your own attack thoughts can just as easily spin around and assault you. This is a major cause of depression, which is a form of self-attack. Anger is a blind emotion with no fixed allegiance. In any form, it is not your friend. It is an enemy to your peace. This is true whether or not anger seems justified in any given circumstance. It is always *you* who will suffer. Make no mistake, anger and attack are the most toxic stuff on earth — and they will never heal on their own. The state of conflict never ends until *you* end it. The only way out of conflict is to recognize its never-ending, brutal nature and then to become dedicated to its opposite.

A secondary but equally important point is that attack and anger need to be corrected at the level of thought. Once this is accomplished, the behavioral issues will fix themselves. To try to heal anger by changing your behavior is like trying to salvage a pot of spoiled stew by adding spices to it. This may cover up the foul taste, but it won't do anything to get rid of the sickening bacteria.

Through experience, you will gradually realize that the gifts of peace far exceed those of attack. Peace is a mightier warrior than attack will ever be, because it reflects our natural state, which means it is immortal. When you give up attack, and by doing so unite with the Spirit of peace, you simultaneously unite in spirit and power with every teacher of peace who has lived, past and present: Mahatma Gandhi, Martin Luther King Jr., Christ, Buddha, Lao Tzu, Paramahansa Yogananda, John Lennon, Mother Teresa, Nelson Mandela, the Dalai Lama, and many, many others. You become one with them, and they with you.

Peace is living manna sent from Heaven, and I have come to believe that it is both the direction and the means of humanity's evolution. Gentleness is strength and defenselessness is the finest armor, because by dedicating your mind to them, you clothe yourself in Spirit and realize that you can never be harmed. You are a part of Spirit, forever, and what you are at your core can never be hurt, killed, or attacked in any way, through any force.

Peace is also the great teacher of meditation. I have watched many meditation students struggle for years with their practice, searching in vain to find the golden key to deep meditation. They search the great teachings, ancient and modern, for that one special technique that they believe will magically transport them into the depths of Great Spirit. Some even go so far as traveling the world, seeking the counsel of sages, priests, and gurus. They sample breathing techniques and learn of ancient Sanskrit mantras, each of which is purported to be the world's most powerful technique. Yet the truth remains that there is only one great teacher of meditation, and we carry that teacher with us every day, everywhere we go, all the time: *choice*.

Gentleness is a choice and nothing more.

Peace, loving-kindness, forgiveness, compassion, unconditional love, gentleness...properly understood, all these teachers are the same, just as the different faces of peace's great human teachers have looked a little different and gone by different names. Christ, Buddha, Martin Luther King Jr., Gandhi — all are one.

It's important to note that self-loathing is also a form of attack. Anger and assault need not be directed outward toward others. As touched on above, you can just as easily attack yourself. Self-contempt, anxiety, depression, guilt, and even many forms of sickness are all examples of self-attacks. You need to learn to love others *and yourself.*

The way to begin cultivating peace is through active forgiveness, gentleness, unconditional love, and all the similar traits. Most people begin this process slowly, experimenting with gentleness a little at a time during their meditations and at moments of obvious conflict. Perhaps, for instance, the next time you are angry with someone, you can try switching your focus from one of blame to one of simple problem solving. Recognize that in most cases your own negative response to a problem is more of an issue than the precipitating problem itself. Blame never helps, and it's always totally unnecessary. *Not blaming* doesn't mean you don't acknowledge problems and work to fix them. For instance, I don't believe that murderers should be allowed to roam the streets. I just think that our correctional system needs to stop focusing on punishing these people and start focusing on healing them. Until that happens, the rate of recidivism will remain obscene, and we will continue getting nowhere fast when it comes to solving the problems of crime and overcrowding in our prison system. Murderers kill because they are locked into hatred. They don't know how to love or even accept love, and until we address this underlying problem, our society will continue to be riddled with violence.

Thankfully, our part in coming to peace is simple. You don't have to fix the correctional facilities of the world, the courts, the governments, or your neighbors. You are responsible only for your own peace, because peace is a personal choice, being an internal state of mind. Begin this process today by recognizing that condemnation in any form accomplishes nothing and generally makes matters worse. Remind yourself every day that you don't want conflict and there is an opposite, which you can choose just as easily. In fact, you can choose peace more easily, because it is a choice that is reinforced by powerful, positive emotions. Once you begin looking at any situation from a problem-solving perspective rather than one of blame, you will see how you can rise above the urge to point fingers and help conflicts to heal instead.

Most important, learn to directly experience the Great Spirit of Peace, which you can glimpse during your meditations. Meditation reinforces peace, and peace reinforces meditation. They are experiences born of one Spirit. From this new perspective, you will come to understand how peace on earth is achieved. It isn't done by changing the world; it is done by changing yourself.

Day 21

For the next ten days, we are going to continue developing our meditative ability using specific techniques, after which our practicing will take a turn toward less specific, more contemplative efforts. For now, these techniques and your experiences with them will provide you with a strong foundation, which will aid you greatly during the less structured exercises to come. As you continue, you will probably find yourself naturally being drawn to one technique more than the others, and you will have the opportunity soon to work with it more intimately, a step that can be of great value.

Speaking of techniques, while we've touched on the chakras that are most often used for meditation (the heart, third eye, and crown), the others can also be used during meditation. Some forms of meditation even use all seven chakras simultaneously, focusing on the energy that flows along the whole system. For reference, the seven chakras, from lowest to highest, are as follows:

1. *Root chakra:* Located at the base of the spine, along the perineum. It is closely associated with baser instincts and individual survival.

2. *Sacral chakra:* Located below the navel. It is most closely associated with sexuality.

3. *Solar plexus chakra:* Located above the navel but below the breastbone. It is the center of ego and individual existence.

4. *Heart chakra:* Located midchest behind the breastbone. It is the center of love, compassion, and higher emotions.

5. *Throat chakra:* Located at the base of the throat where the left and right collarbones meet in a V. It is associated with communication, whether verbal or nonverbal.

6. *Third eye chakra:* Located between the eyebrows. It is thought to be the hub of spiritual sight and intuition.

7. *Crown chakra:* Located at the top of the head. It is generally considered to be the seat of the higher self.

For practical applications, think of the chakras as existing in a straight line that runs directly up the spinal column from the base of your spine and your perineum to the top of your head. Today's meditation uses all seven.

First, after you are settled and relaxed, spend a brief time placing your attention on each chakra, beginning at the lowest and moving upward to the crown. Spend no more than a minute or so on each one, tuning in your mind to each point while trying to sense the energy there. If you have difficulties focusing on any one in particular or feel an unusual amount of tension or other odd physical sensations, this is thought to indicate a block in the energy flow. The common interpretation of such blocks is that you may have certain lessons to learn in relation to that particular form of chakra energy. For instance:

- A block at the root chakra might indicate issues with security and trust.

- Sacral chakra blocks are linked to sexuality and associated feelings of guilt.

- Solar plexus blocks are linked with humility, giving, and selflessness issues.

- Blocks at the heart chakra are linked with challenges in learning to give and receive love, show compassion, and forgive others.

- Throat chakra blocks are linked with difficulties in open communication, which also involve intimacy and trust themes.

- Third eye blocks may indicate struggles with intuition and nonphysical insight.

- And blocks at the crown chakra concern the development of spiritual trust and releasing the fear of loss of ego identity.

If you experience any feelings of obstructed energy, take note of the particular chakra involved and the associated feeling, whether it is a tingling or other odd sensation, numbness, inability to concentrate well, or something else, and then move on to the next chakra until you have meditated on each one. If it helps, you might imagine a glowing crystal at each chakra, thus having an image to guide your focus. When you are done, spend the remainder of your meditation focusing on simple relaxation. You will use your experiences today during tomorrow's exercise.

Day 22

Yesterday's meditation was intended to reveal areas that need development in you, for we stand to develop most dramatically through working on our weaknesses. With today's meditations, think back to your experience yesterday. Identify the chakra that gave you the most trouble or produced unusual feelings or tension, and take a moment to review yesterday's notes regarding that chakra.

Then spend a few minutes during the beginning of your meditation today considering how that chakra plays a part in your daily life and relationships, and how it may be affecting you negatively. For instance, consider how sexual guilt interferes with giving and receiving love; how a lack of trust in life leads to fear, which leads to our being closed off and guarded; how problems with communication cause misunderstandings and may hold us back on many levels, such as professionally and in our relationships; and so on. Just let your thoughts roam randomly in this manner. Also note any parallels between the chakra in question and your life and personality as they are today.

Finally, focus your attention on the chakra in question, and imagine it as if it were a small sphere composed of pure energy, joined to the other chakras by a thin, flowing ribbon of light running up and down the spinal column. Ideally, the chakras should not be closed off from each other, like discrete lakes, but should instead be part of an open system that feeds directly from one point to the next, like a series of lakes connected by rivers. In this exercise, you are attempting to open up this system and stimulate the flow. You may wish to combine this concentration exercise with one of the key words associated with it from Day 21. For instance, if you are working on the root chakra, direct your attention to the base of your spine while repeating the word "*safe*" or "*peace*" with each exhalation.

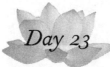

Day 23

Today, turn your focus to the whole system of chakras as if it were a single, linked system of energy — that is, as if there were only one chakra, not seven. Today's meditation combines a chakra meditation with a visualization exercise.

After you are relaxed, begin by imagining a small ball of light moving up and down your spinal column among the seven chakras, from the root chakra to the crown chakra and then back down again. Try to feel the energy of the chakra system building, as if the movement of the ball of light were causing the system to polarize, pulling your attention deeper and deeper inward. Link the movement to your breath so that the ball ascends during your inhalations and descends during each out-breath. Think of this exercise as being intended to liberate the energy flow along this pathway, and feel it growing stronger, more free-flowing, and smoother with each cycle.

Day 24

As you no doubt have noticed, meditative techniques can be combined to form unique exercises, such as yesterday's practice. Today's lesson is another great example of this method. Furthermore, today's meditation cuts straight to the fundamental purpose of the techniques involved — visualization, mantra, and chakra meditation — by focusing directly on the development of peace through forgiveness.

After you are relaxed, pick one person from your life toward whom you have unhealed anger. You are going to use this person and your grievances with them in an attempt to touch, if only faintly, the release that forgiveness can bring. It doesn't matter whom you choose, but don't explicitly exclude any particular person because you believe your feelings about them are too harsh. The first person who comes to mind will work well enough.

Since the heart chakra is the one most closely associated with forgiveness, begin your meditation by focusing on it. Anchor your mind on the heart chakra; then, with each in-breath, imagine that there is a light in your chest that is growing just a little bit brighter, and with each exhalation, imagine that the light is growing a little bit larger. Inhaling, brighter; exhaling, larger; inhaling, brighter; exhaling, larger. Focus on this dynamic visualization for a few minutes until the light has spread throughout your body and formed a cocoon surrounding it. This is your real protection. Within this cocoon, you are safe and at peace.

Next, imagine the person you have chosen for the purpose of this exercise sitting directly in front of you. Quietly regard them, and briefly consider the two or three main points of conflict between you. What hurts most? Don't dwell on this part for long, and don't allow yourself to get caught up in sorrow, betrayal, or anger. Just calmly recall your major points of contention.

Finally, imagine yourself telling the person,

> *As I forgive you for your mistakes,*
> *I forgive myself for mine. I choose to do so now,*
> *so that we both may know peace and joy together.*

Repeat this over and over again like a mantra, thoughtfully and with as much sincerity as you can muster. Spend at least several minutes on this practice, seeking the key to making forgiveness real to you. Notice how the farther you are able to go in the direction of forgiveness, the deeper and more powerful your experience becomes.

For your evening meditation, choose someone else as your focus, repeating the same procedures outlined above.

Day 25

Meditation is not limited to the practices we have been sampling thus far. There are numerous types of meditation, including moving meditations like yoga and tai chi; meditations to music; guided meditations, which sometimes include elaborate visual imagery; and contemplations. It isn't the purpose of this book to cover all of these and the many other styles out there. Exploration of techniques can be helpful to a point; however, its use is limited in the long run.

Replacing negative thoughts with happiness, self-acceptance, peace, appreciation, compassion, forgiveness, and joy is what will ultimately take you deeper into your practicing. If the techniques you are using during your meditations are not facilitating this, their use is limited. This is why the words, thoughts, and images I have selected for these exercises have been carefully chosen.

Today, our focus will be on joy. As you begin, ask yourself silently, "What is joy?" and then try to reach inward and sense the presence of joy within you, rather than allowing mere words to provide an answer. True joy is a pure state that arises from our core self as we release our judgments, which means it is always present in our lives. Our attention is shifted away from joy when we try seeking it in the world outside of us. True joy isn't based merely on pleasant worldly circumstances and experiences. If it were, it would be fickle indeed. It is not something we make, define, or achieve. It is something we embrace and accept.

Try today to experience the natural joy that radiates from within you as you sink down quietly into your inner self. Just sit quietly, and become perfectly still and at peace. If your mind wanders, repeat the question "What is joy?" several times if need be, until you feel your mind quieting down.

Also, try to sense the feeling of safety that comes with joy, the satisfaction it brings, and the generalized feeling that everything is going to be okay. In Spirit, you are safe. You are healed. You are whole. You are at peace.

Day 26

Another helpful meditation tool, especially useful for beginners, is meditation music and recordings of other peaceful sounds, such as those of nature, gongs, and singing bowls. If you are having difficulty disciplining yourself to sit down and meditate regularly, putting on light background music can be helpful. The right choice of music can instill a sense of peace, just as a good mantra is intended to do. There are many recordings geared toward meditation, and they can be either purchased as CDs or downloaded from the Internet. Or you can use any peaceful music that suits you. Just remember that while using music, the object is still to stay focused on your meditation and not on the music.

For something different, set the mood for your meditations today by putting on some background music. Use yesterday's meditation once more, focusing on tapping into the sense of inner joy, even if it is very faint.

Day 27

So far, we have experimented with zazen, mantra, visualization, chakra, and meditations designed to elicit feelings of forgiveness. Besides these, there are some types of meditation that are a little subtler, like the one you've used over the past two days, which focuses on the idea of joy.

Mindfulness, which is a type of zazen, is another popular style of meditation. This ancient Buddhist practice — said to have been handed down directly from the original Buddha, Siddhartha Gautama, sometime around 500 BCE — can take many forms, but by far the most common is mindfulness of the breath.

To practice, begin as usual, and then adopt a calm awareness of the breathing process. That is, tune in to the sensations surrounding the respiratory cycle. To be mindful really just means *to pay attention to*. So try to experience your breath directly, sensing the air moving in and out, in and out, while gently maintaining a single-pointed focus on this function. Sense the natural rhythm of the breathing cycle, which fills your body with life and is so perfectly aligned with nature. Like the tides of the sea, which go in and out daily in a natural cycle, so too is your breath aligned with the rhythm of life.

Alternatively, you can focus your attention on the sensation of air flowing past the tips of your nostrils, feeling it drawing in cool and coming out warm:

Inhaling, cool; exhaling, warm;
inhaling, cool; exhaling, warm.

During this practice, the breath should not be forced, manipulated, or controlled in any way but should be allowed to flow naturally. You should be focusing only on your awareness of the process, or on the feeling of air passing back and forth across the threshold of your nostrils. And just as with other meditations, as you are *tuning in* to today's focus, you should be simultaneously *tuning out* distracting thoughts.

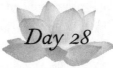

Day 28

Another common mindfulness technique involves the practice of maintaining an awareness of the physical body. The idea is to acquire a firm, though calm, awareness of being at one with your body. Sense the powerful life force that links you to your body, feel its presence, and allow this awareness to become the focus of your meditation.

At first, this exercise may seem to run counter to the basic meditative objective of moving beyond bodily awareness; however, as you practice it with intensity, you'll find that this is not the case. As with any single-pointed focus, the more you concentrate on it to the exclusion of everything else, the nearer you come to the present, which is the gateway to meditative peace. We'll talk in detail soon about the present moment and how it applies to meditation. We've already said that during any meditation, you are moving inward, away from the physical. What we haven't gotten into deeply just yet is that you are also moving away from the past and future, and into the present. In the case of mindfulness of the body, by becoming highly present in your immediate physical self, you reduce the mind's temporal projections as well. The spiritual phrase "Be here now," which was popularized by the 1971 book of the same title by Ram Dass, means to become aware of your immediate existence in this precise moment of time. However, focusing on only one of these objectives automatically brings an immediate awareness of the other, since time and space are not separate. Therefore, if you are aware of the *now*, you also become aware of the immediate *here* by extension — and vice versa. They are only different points of view of the same phenomenon.

Begin today's meditation by tensing and relaxing your body

several times as you inhale and exhale deeply, feeling energy surge and diminish throughout your body, and then relax fully and let your breathing return to normal. Now try to sense your connection with your body directly. Get a feel for being firmly seated within it and for the powerful life presence at your core. Feel this not as a thought but as a direct experience, and do not allow other thoughts to intrude and pull you away from this awareness. Mindfulness is about direct awareness, which should not be confused with thought or interpretations of the experience. The lack of interpretation is what makes mindfulness what it is.

Day 29

In our recent meditations, we have been transitioning from practicing with explicit techniques to doing less-structured meditation. Today's practice will be one more step in this direction. In the meditative tradition often called *just sitting*, the practitioner is given no mantra, visualization, or other focus. This style of meditation is as simple as it sounds. It is a free form, the idea being to simply allow thoughts to come and go without any involvement with them.

To begin, close your eyes, get settled as usual, and then relax inward. Your thoughts will start coming and going instantly; however, just as with other forms of meditative practice, allow no particular thought to grab your attention and begin weaving a web of thoughts to entrap you. Instead, merely watch each one rise in your mind, take note of it, and then let it disappear like a leaf being swept away by a steady wind. Another thought will quickly take its place, of course, and another, and another, and so on. As each one comes to mind, follow the same procedure outlined above. That is, let it come without fighting it, notice it, and then allow it to slip away into the oblivion from which it came. Above all else, do not allow yourself to be drawn into a continuing internal dialogue. This process is to be repeated throughout the meditative session, with the only focus being a sensation of growing inner peace.

Essentially, during *just sitting*, you are doing exactly that. Sit down, become as calm and quiet as you can, and let your mind be at peace for a little while.

Day 30

Today's emphasis will be similar to yesterday's. There will be no particular technique to use, no central focus. Instead, try to allow yourself to relax into an ever-deepening sense of peace. Feel as if you are sinking inward toward the center of your mind, toward its core. For this, it is important to understand that you don't need to do anything at all. The mind naturally turns inward when we stop interfering and just let go. Without your interference, your constant thoughts and emphasis and physical sensations, you would instantly connect with your core self, just as a heavy weight tossed into a pool sinks to the bottom. All you need to do is relax and learn the art of just letting go.

PART THREE

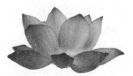

REPROGRAMMING
THE WATERFALL

Introduction

Today our journey together takes a turn. Now we are shifting our focus from technique to the deepening of our connection with core self by changing our internal programming just a bit, day by day.

The daily thoughts and exercises contained in the following meditations are powerful tools that you will want to use not only during your formal meditations but anytime you need more peace or are searching for guidance and connection with your core self. Each exercise begins with a thought of the day, which you might consider a little nugget of truth intended for quiet reflection. The more you think these thoughts, the more you work with them and make them an everyday part of your life, the more thoroughly you will assimilate them. This will result in deeper meditations during your formal practicing, as well as profound changes in how you deal with the circumstances of your life and the people who share it with you. After all, meditation will do you little practical good if it doesn't help you in daily life too, which is where we face most of our challenges to peace.

In a sense, during part 3 of this book, we are becoming more concerned with the *content* of our meditations and less with their form. During your meditations, use the daily thoughts as *focus sentences*. In some cases, instructions will be given as to how you should apply the focus sentence during practice; but in general, you should repeat the idea several times slowly and with intention at the beginning of your meditations, considering its meaning along with the thoughts that accompany it. Then simply try, using whatever technique appeals to you, to sink down into deep stillness and peace. You may utilize any of the meditative techniques that were presented in part 2, if you wish, or no particular technique at all. Let your intuition be your guide as to which technique, if any, to use, but keep in mind that you should not allow your mind to wander randomly. Keep your focus on your meditation. If you become distracted, repeat the focus sentence again, several times if need be, and then return to the attempt to let peace envelop you.

As mentioned above, you can bring the daily thoughts to mind and repeat them mentally any time you feel the need, and even when you don't feel any particular need. Try to remember them as often as possible, and when you have time, pause for a minute or even less, close your eyes, and repeat them to yourself. Think of them as medicine for your mind. They aren't meant to replace your thoughts but rather to begin reprogramming your waterfall of thoughts so that all of them will one day reflect peace.

Opening to the Mystical Moment

The mystical moment originates in the here and now. You can ac-cess it only by merging your entire being into the present, even if this awareness lasts for an instant.

There is a moment that can be achieved through meditation that is so perfect, so healing and enchanting, it is unlike anything you have ever experienced before. Nothing in our world compares to it. Opening up to this perfect moment puts you in touch with a Power mighty enough to instantly change the direction of your life at the most fundamental level.

This instant is what I call the *mystical moment*, although there are other names for it, such as *holy instant*, *mystical experience*, and so on. Once again, as with the terms *God* and *core self*, what you call it does not matter. What does matter is that the experience of the mystical moment is exactly the same for everyone, regardless of religion, nationality, race, individual beliefs, personality, or any other stratifying ego characteristics. It is an experience of coming into full, conscious contact with your core self, and it occurs as we release our focus on the past and future and become totally absorbed in the present.

Although impossible to describe in words, the mystical moment is saturated with joy. It is the purest form of joy that we, as human beings, are capable of. It is our highest, most exalted state. The more of your life that you spend in the presence of the mystical moment, the freer you will be, the more joy you will experience, and the more personal power you will command.

I could go on and on describing the mystical moment to you, but since it needs to be experienced in order to be comprehended, the wiser course is to point out the conditions through which it is achieved, rather than dwelling on what can never be expressed. Only the blocks to the experience — which exist solely in the mind — hinder your awareness of the mystical moment. Once these blocks are released, the mystical moment is instantly experienced, because it is *always present*.

Pause and reflect on that for a moment. The mystical moment is with you now. The only reason why you may be unaware of it is that your attention is focused elsewhere — in memories of the past or anticipations of the future. To experience the mystical moment, you need do nothing more than pause your own mental projections into the past and future. That is, you temporarily stop thinking about anything that has to do with either past or future. The mystical moment's eternal presence will then become readily apparent to you.

Projection of thought into the past and future is the primary obstacle to the mystical moment. In fact, it is the only obstacle. This must be true, because the present is the only time there really is. This is not a curious philosophical speculation. It is an observable fact. While your mind is engaged in the past and future, you are dwelling in a fantasy realm because the past and future do not have any current reality. We touched on this earlier, but now we will consider it more carefully.

It isn't too difficult to see that the present moment is the only aspect of time that is real. Think of the past, for instance. Clearly, it is gone and exists only in your memory. By definition, the past has already elapsed. It isn't something you can change, touch, or act in. You cannot hold it in your hand, but just in wisps of flimsy, ever-shifting memory. Your only real power regarding the past is in how you choose to *interpret* it right now. Yet even this involves a present choice.

Regarding the future, it is equally unreal as you regard it from your present perspective. You can anticipate it from afar, but as it unfurls and suddenly manifests in your present life, it is no longer the future. Once again, this is true by definition, since the future is commonly defined as *time yet to come*. When it does show up, it instantly morphs into your present reality. The only thing that makes time seem concrete is that it appears to be accompanied by change. However, if the temporal progression is not real, what must that imply about the world we live in and the changes we seem to experience?

In actuality, you can never exist outside of the present moment. Even if you are unaware of the here and now, your existence remains tied to it. When you choose to anchor your mind to the present, all you are doing is choosing to acknowledge your own reality. The only choice we ever face, then — and we do so in each instant of our lives — is whether to focus and use the incredible power of our minds to shape our reality through the present, or, instead, to expend that creative energy building a fantasyland in our heads.

Projections into the past and future go on all the time. Most of us are never aware of this process, and so we spend precious little time with a mind clear of past thoughts and future concerns. As your meditation practice continues to deepen and evolve, however, you will begin to see just how powerful and liberating keeping to the present can be.

The practice of dwelling in the present is not only about achieving transcendent, mystical awareness. It is also about attaining simple peace of mind. Doing so frees you from judgments about the past, grievances and anger over what others have done, guilt over what you have done, and fear and uncertainty over what your future holds. On the simplest level, this alleviates stress and therefore promotes the health of both mind and body. It is impossible to experience anxiety, depression, anger, or guilt while you are focused on the present moment, since these emotions always involve some projection either forward or backward in time — into what has already gone by or what is yet to be.

On a more profound level, minding the moment opens you up to the miraculous energy that forms the foundation of every cell of your body, every feeling that surges through you, every thought that you think — that is, the energy of Source. By aligning yourself with the present moment, you align with core self; and by extension, you open a direct channel for Source energy to come into your life. This energy is capable of producing fundamental shifts in your consciousness — and even, at times, in your life circumstances. It is not limited. As it spreads outward from Source and through your life, it holds the potential to heal you at every level, whether emotional, circumstantial, or physical.

Meditation tunes you in to the here and now, and unlocks the miraculous power contained in the mystical moment — the most intense experience of the present. The mystical moment comes to you when you have fully released yourself to the present and realize in full awareness your identity as core self.

When you meditate, try to let go of all thoughts about the past, regardless of their nature, as well as all future concerns. Also, keep in mind that it doesn't matter whether thoughts regarding the past and future are judged to be positive or negative, happy or sad, important or trivial. To tap into the present moment, you must let go of *all* thoughts about what's gone by and what's to come, and actively focus only on your here and now.

You will find that with practice, dwelling in the present moment is easier than you might imagine, and it will bring you a new form of joy not available in any fantasy. So take time for the only real time there is. The present is always with you. But where are you?

Day 31

In this perfect moment, I am perfect within my core self.
I am safe, I am whole, I am healed, I am complete.

Our first thought of the day begins with a reflection on the present moment, core self, and the feeling of safety and peace that communion with core self brings. When we dwell only in the present, we automatically become aware of our core self, which is perfect, complete, at peace, and forever safe. This is a point we have made before, and will make again and again. It is so important that it cannot be considered too often. The more often you remind yourself of the perfect immutability of your core self, the safer, and hence more at peace, you will feel.

To review, it is by relinquishing all thoughts of past and future concerns that we open to the present and learn that the ego and the body are just limited, temporary expressions of core self, like ripples on the ocean. They are not you. You are the ocean itself, but when you identify with the ripples only, you forget your true nature.

Use the thought of the day as a focus sentence, repeating it several times slowly at the beginning of your meditations today and again whenever you feel the need to refocus. Also, take a minute to repeat it just before you end your practice, thinking about the words and what they mean. Most important, try to feel the deeper truth that the words point to. What you are is not for words to say, but they can point you in the right direction. Unless otherwise specified, this is how you should use all the following thoughts of the day during your meditations.

As already mentioned, in the main body of your meditations,

you may also choose to use one of the specific meditation techniques introduced in part 2 after you have considered the focus sentence. This will be up to you, but it is especially encouraged for beginners. The use of words, images, and other specific meditations can be highly useful during the initial training period. At a minimum, be sure to use the thought of the day whenever needed to help you stay focused.

Day 32

The mystical moment is always present.
To find it, I need do nothing but let go,
release all thoughts of past and future,
and sink peacefully into the here and now.

The mystical moment is always with you. In fact, every moment can be a mystical moment. There is a misconception that a great deal of time and an exorbitant amount of practice are needed to learn how to experience it, but this cannot be true, because the mystical moment is nothing more than a temporary *relinquishment of time.* This is precisely why it requires nothing more significant than a *lack of effort.* Can a lack of effort possibly be conceived of as being difficult or taking a long time to accomplish? Only the ego would have us believe so.

It is equally important to realize that the mystical moment can never be found in the future. The belief that you will somehow be better able to accomplish it later — another day, another year, another lifetime — is one of the primary ego defenses against it. Be determined in your meditations to find the mystical moment right where it is, *within you,* and right when it is — *now!* Now is an eternal state, not a future one.

You don't have to be a meditation master to commune with the present. You don't need to have years of experience. The mystical moment is open to everyone, of all levels of experience, because it is where our core self exists, and so it is our reality. Become determined to let go of all thoughts related to both the past and future, and become perfectly centered in the present and grounded in your *immediate* practice. Sink into the present by letting go of all thoughts not relating to the here and now, and don't allow your ego to tell you that you can find the present only in the future. Clearly this stance makes absolutely no sense. The present can be found only in the present, which obviously cannot be far away. It is always right where you are, and right when you are.

Day 33

One instant is all I need to give. I offer it now.

I often share today's thought with students who come to my workshops. Don't try to make your whole meditation perfect. Just try to make *one instant* of it perfect. Ask yourself if you are capable of giving just one instant fully. The closer you come to doing so, the more powerful your experiences will become. For just as the mystical moment can never be found in the future, only one instant is needed to experience it fully.

Yesterday I pointed out that finding the present moment does not require time. Today's idea takes this thought one step further. One instant given fully to the here and now, backed by whole-hearted desire, is enough to draw you directly into it. This happens quite naturally, since the present moment is our natural state, and it is where your core self exists already. It doesn't require you to attain some exalted, impossible-to-reach state. You only need to let go of everything else, everything that blocks your awareness of it. All the intruding thoughts and beliefs, the extra stuff we have added on to our core self, are what clutters our minds and makes the mystical moment seem difficult to find.

Forget about trying to make your entire meditation perfect, transcendent, and blissful — whether it is five minutes or ten or twenty. Aim to give everything you've got to letting go and connecting to core self for just a fraction of a second. For just one moment, release all notions you have about life, God, who and what you are; all judgments from the past and all concerns over the future; and everything else not pertaining to the moment at hand. For just *one instant*, put all your effort into your practice, and you will see how powerful such super-focused efforts can be. Remember, as suggested in the beginning of this book, it is not the quantity of meditation that matters but the quality. Make just one instant count, and that perfect instant will draw you back again and again, becoming a reference point you can rely on, just as a sailor may learn how to use the North Star to navigate the world's seas once he identifies its position in the sky.

Day 34

*Right now is the only time I am free to choose
what I want my future to be, and I do so
by choosing what I want this moment to be.
Peace, joy, and freedom from fear are one choice.*

Read through today's thought a few times, memorize it, and make sure you understand this idea fully. It is a powerful notion that can change your life forever, if only it is understood and embraced. When you practice meditating on the present moment, try thinking of each instant as all there is to time — the only dimension with any reality. Try to realize that fundamentally there is no past and no future but only the here and now. You cannot choose to be happy and at peace in the future, and likewise you cannot change anything that has already occurred in the past. You can, however, decide what your present state of mind should be, and it is this, and only this, that empowers you to shape your future. Whatever you want to feel in the future, decide to feel it *now* and keep your mind focused on it. In this way, you will experience it immediately and carry it with you as you move through time.

Peace has always been, and will forever be, a present choice. There is no other path to peace beyond this simple, logical realization. *Present* peace of mind can be achieved only through *present* choice. And so it is with future peace, since there is no future beyond mental extrapolations. Choose peace now, fully, and you will see it cover your past, present, and future alike.

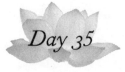

Day 35

I rest in stillness.

Just as clouds can look like thick, solid objects from the ground, yet an airplane can pass straight through them unencumbered, so too can your thoughts appear deceptively compelling. The only power they have to distract you and keep you "grounded" during meditation is whatever power you give them. In reality, they are just passing, wispy dreams blowing across the surface of your mind, like clouds moving with the wind, shifting, changing shape, disappearing and reappearing, darkening from white to gray to black and lightening again. Let them all come and go as they will, but don't imagine that they have any more power to hold you back than a cloud has to stop a pigeon's flight.

And so it is with your own mind. Internal space calls you constantly, and your thoughts cannot hold you back. You can choose to ride their currents, becoming stuck in them, or you can choose to let them go and to move through them and beyond them. They are nothing more than shifting forms composed of nothingness. You have been watching these shapes move across the screen of your mind for your entire life. Wouldn't you like to see the land that lies beyond them?

Instead of becoming absorbed with this restless old picture show today, relax into the stillness beyond your thoughts, in which a much more interesting experience awaits you. It is an ancient experience, far older than anything on earth, including your personal thoughts. It is an experience of the timeless self within you. Seek only this experience during today's meditations, and let your thoughts pass by without interest. Any that are important will still be there when you are done meditating. You can attend to them later.

Rest your mind! Rest your body! Rest deeply today! Tell yourself as often as you wish, both during your meditations and in between as well,

I rest in stillness.

The more you remind yourself of this, the better. And you can have nothing to fear by resting. As will be discussed later, in the chapter titled "Health and Healing," both your body and your mind will only be fortified by your efforts to let go and abandon ego for a while. Feel how deep, how restful, and how rejuvenating meditation can be — how much your mind and spirit have been longing for this rest. Be kind to your mind and rest it today; and be kind to your body as well, and rest it too. Go as deeply as you can into the stillness within, and be at peace for a little while.

*Let me see this moment in the light of the present
instead of the shadow of the past.*

The past is a veil that blinds us to our current reality, obscuring and coloring everything we see and experience, along with everyone we meet. Because of this, while we are relying on the past as our guide, we never see anything with true clarity. We see, instead, only shadows of the true world, mixed up with a conglomeration of our own projected images. In contrast, the present moment is crystal clear and beautiful to dwell in. There is a sublime perfection in it, and as you give it a space in your life, it will surround you with a sense of peace and safety. The present is quiet and very still; subtle and yet powerful; transforming but forever steady, forever present, and completely unwavering. The past, which typically emphasizes judgment, strips away the beauty of the present and imprisons us in a world of shadows and dreams, unshared thoughts, and imagination. It builds a wall that you cannot see beyond and makes life seem dulled, lifeless, and dreamlike, like the past itself. The present is pure joy; the past, absolute imprisonment. The present is liberation; the past, leaden with sorrow.

The only thoughts from the past that easily translate to present joy are the memories of happiness you have shared with other people. These thoughts reflect a union that transcends the past, and so these gentle thoughts are not our major concern. Most of the past thoughts we tend to focus on are thoughts about how others have hurt us or how we have hurt them — in other words, attack thoughts that are directed either toward others or toward ourselves. It doesn't truly matter which, for both types are equally disruptive to present peace.

Look at your past as if it were nothing more than a passing movie that has little, if any, bearing on your current life. Liberate yourself from the wounds of the past, whether they were inflicted by you or by another, and you will begin to see the world around you through brand-new eyes. These are baby eyes, which don't judge and always see truly. Only forgiveness of the past, which is the opposite of judgment, makes this exchange possible.

Day 37

*In this perfect moment I have no outside needs.
I am fulfilled by direct contact with my core self.*

t is impossible to explain to those who have never tried it that by letting go of all other thoughts, wants, and needs, we actually *gain*. We are all seeking satisfaction, fulfillment, and happiness. The trouble is, we are looking in the wrong places. We try to fulfill ourselves through things and experiences of all kinds and shapes — alcohol, food, sex, money, fame, shopping, power, praise, drugs, achievements, and many other forms. Yet none of these things will ever satisfy our restless souls. You can try as many forms as you like, for as long as you like, but none of them will ever bring you lasting satisfaction.

That said, it's important to be clear that seeking fulfillment in the external world is not evil. It's not a "sin." This is where a lot of people become confused. They think that seeking worldly pleasure is either evil or pleasurable, but few realize that it is neither — it is neutral, except that while we are doing so, we tend to ignore the richness of the spiritual world that is within us.

By releasing your fixation on external gratification, you will discover the intense inner satisfaction that derives from your core self. The reason why communing with core self is so satisfying is that — even though we don't often realize it — we all crave this experience of union with our true self. Without an active, open awareness of this deepest, primal connection, we are walking about in this world only half alive, and a part of us senses it. We do realize on some level that a major part of our life is missing, and it is this hole that causes us to constantly crave, crave,

crave. This is why people overeat. They are trying to fill up with food the vacant space they sense inside themselves; it is also why alcoholics drink themselves into oblivion over and over and over again. They think that one more drink will somehow, magically, satisfy them. Yet this is no great crime. It is an error, no doubt about it, because it doesn't work. But there is no evil intent behind it. We are all looking to fill the emptiness we think exists within us.

The truth is, there is no emptiness within you. You can find fulfillment only by reconnecting with core self. I am not suggesting that you need to focus on changing your behavior. You don't need to make any major changes to the external circumstances of your life to reconnect with your core self, but you do need to begin looking the right direction — inward. Morning and night today, practice making this connection by putting aside all the things you think you want, and even the things you think you need, and instead seek only one thing: inner connection with your core. It is this connection that will satisfy you and bring you peace. Try to sense how the closer you come to your core, the more your sense of satisfaction increases; and notice how your feeling of satisfaction dissipates as you let your mind stray to outside thoughts, objects, and objectives. Get a sense of the contrast that can be felt between external seeking and internal seeking.

You don't need to give up the things of the world, but just to shift your priorities a little during your meditations. What you find will be far more convincing than anything I have to say about this matter. Experience is life's greatest teacher.

*As I release the future, I am freed from anxiety
over future uncertainties and dreams to come.
In the present moment, I am liberated from fear.*

As has been suggested, the future, like the past, easily becomes an obstacle to deep meditation, and a major breeding ground for fear. When we fixate on what's to come in the future, we often become paralyzed by anxiety or else thoroughly occupied with planning. This is an obvious impediment to present peace.

During today's meditations, watch your mind for any thoughts about the future, and be sure to redirect yourself away from them, releasing your future so that you can come alive in the present. While we focus on the future, we are never truly alive in the present. We cannot be fully conscious of everything we are in the here and now while we are committing any part of our mind to some unreal future state. Doing so always robs us of present peace and gives us nothing in return. You can never fully control or predict the future. In this world, there are far too many unpredictable variables. The best we can do is aim our life in a *general direction* for future growth. Yet even this, as has been pointed out, is a matter of a present, conscious decision.

During meditation, and even as an exercise at any time during the day, try letting each moment stand out fresh and new, independent of both past and future. Surround each instant with a tiny sacred space that is free from fear, free from judgment, and free from all uncertainties about what your future will bring, cannot bring, or *should* bring in order to make you happy. When you let go of the future in this way, you are acknowledging that you do not know what's best, and as you cease constantly trying to plan out your future, you open up a space in which the will of Source can enter and introduce undreamed-of possibilities into your life. Thus, things you never could have planned for are given the room they need to occur. As you release both your dreams and your fears for the future, you are letting go of the steering wheel of your life and allowing your future to become part of a much greater cosmic plan of awakening — one so vast that no human could ever conceive of its design. Don't bother trying. Even if you could, there is no need. The same Intelligence that brought you, and all life, into being still resides within you. It didn't need your help to give you life, and it does not need your help to make your future meaningful. Just stop interfering by trying to control things on your own, and you will see how great, brilliant, and joyous your life can become.

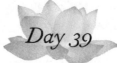

Day 39

More than anything else,
I want to remember my core self.

Your core self does not ask much from you in order to bring you peace and healing. In fact, it requires only one thing, which is absolutely essential. It asks that you love it and want to experience it above anything else — at least for one perfect instant. Your own sincere desire, in your command alone, is the only force that can rejoin your awareness with your core, because desire is the active agent of the single most powerful thing in the physical universe — *your will*.

Will is the force that shapes your entire life, and when you really want something, your will cannot help but bring it to you. This is as true of negative experiences as it is of positive ones. It may be something you have wanted only unconsciously, or even something you don't want at all but believe you deserve, such as sickness, but either way, the power of your will is still in full effect. The world we live in is like the holodeck from the series *Star Trek*. You program it beforehand, step inside, and immerse yourself in a lifelike, fictional realm where what you want and believe fuses with the power of your will and — *poof!* — comes to life. Most people never even realize this is happening, because they have immersed themselves so deeply in the dream of physical time and space that they can no longer remember their core self at all, which is where the power of will originates. They don't see that they are shaping their own destiny. Instead, all they are able to see now is the outside world, which seems to be the cause of what they experience. Yet the outside world is nothing more than a reflection of the inside world. If, then, the power of your will lies asleep in unconsciousness, the world itself seems to become your master. It binds and traps you in its web, becoming the only home you can remember. Furthermore, since it is a world that appears to exist completely independent of your will, you will believe you are powerless against it.

Use today's idea to communicate to your core self your desire to remember your true home and, by doing so, to remember your own native power. The power of your will is still with you even now, though you appear to be cut off from it. Call to it; long for it; give it your attention, your desire, and your love; and most important, turn inward toward it. Repeat today's idea many times during your meditations, slowly, while trying to sense your core, and remember that peace and quietness of thought are the keys to opening that connection.

Day 40

*Right now, in this mystical moment,
I am at peace with all aspects of life.
I am at one with my core self, my mind, and my body.*

Use each of our daily thoughts to bring you a sense of peace and balance, and be sure to apply them directly to any thought you find particularly disturbing. It is the unhealed parts of your life — the conflicts, uncertainties, guilt, judgments, and fears — that disrupt meditation most profoundly. However, negative thoughts not only affect your practice. They also affect you in many other ways, even when you are not aware of them.

As you practice with today's idea, try to gain a sense of letting it ease any unhealed conflicts. You will gradually discover that conflict is an inner state, no matter how much it seems to come from external forces, situations, and other people. If realizing this seems difficult to you, a rudimentary lesson might begin with the simple realization that at the very least, our own negative reactions to external difficulties often exacerbate things, and so we would certainly be better off if we learned to respond to life's challenges in a way that didn't make them worse.

Let your meditations become a place where you go to find comfort and safety from the endless problems of the external world. There is no end to them, and they come in all varieties, sizes, and forms. You can only do your best to deal with each one as it pops up, realizing that more will certainly follow. That's life on earth, but don't let this depress you. Instead, try to realize how you can be safe inside your own mind from external influences if you so choose. You can cultivate a space of peace within you

so stable that no external nightmare can shake it. This is not es-
capism. Temporarily going beyond life's difficulties will help you
to resolve them much more effectively. By quieting your mind,
you will gain the ability to think more clearly, recognize how you
contribute to your own problems, and also see how you can more
easily solve many of them instead of using them to preserve ego.
This attitude alone is valuable beyond any worldly treasure. It is
the difference between defensiveness and empowerment, stag-
nation and growth, and dreaming of time and awakening to the
present.

The Key to Emotional Balance

Growing up spiritually involves much more than taking responsibility for your behavior. It requires you to do so at an infinitely more fundamental level — the level of thought.

Within each of us, a war is being waged. It is a battle that goes on all the time, every day, in every human being who has ever set foot on this planet. It is the struggle between the desire to be a separate entity with an independent will and existence, and the reality of our nature, which is one of perfect, unbroken union.

We are not separate from each other or our Source, even though in this world we seem to be. We appear to be separated from others by our bodies, which keep us locked into narrow physical prisons, alone and held apart from other people. During deep meditation, you can sense your connection with others as your awareness reaches inward beyond the physical realm, back into the collective consciousness of humanity. This is the reason why the body can never make separation real. Our connection together is an internal one, and nothing outside of us has any power to divide what is one by its nature. The body itself is just a tiny vehicle you can use to look out upon and interact with the external world, but it isn't really a prison. Looking through its eyes is like looking through a peephole in a door. Through it, you see only what is outside, on the other side of the door. If you become transfixed in this position, you may even begin to believe that the world on the other side of the door is all there is to life. Yet turn around and you will find that you are living in a luxurious mansion of comfort, peace, and unassailable safety. This is meditation's grandest vision.

To struggle against our unity is both painful and exhausting, since it involves the continuous denial of our reality. Imagine if you really were stuck standing at a door, keeping your eye pressed against the peephole. This would quickly become exhausting, and your view would be significantly limited. Yet this is precisely what we are doing by looking at life exclusively through the body's eyes. The body can see only what is outside of us, and thus its viewpoint is fundamentally limited.

The process of viewing life solely through the body's eyes is not only exhausting and limited but also a wasted effort. However, it is such a pervasive viewpoint in our world for a reason. Buried deep down in the human psyche is a thick layer of guilt that fuels a vicious psychological struggle. This layer of guilt is the root cause of much of our suffering. It causes us at various moments to feel miserable about ourselves, tired, helpless, depressed, anxious, and even physically ill. It also triggers an intense internal fear, which is the fundamental reason why most people tend to stay so thoroughly focused on the external. We believe that our inner core is tainted by guilt, and so we have, in effect, become afraid of what we really are.

This guilt and fear fuels what I call the *guilt cycle*. Even if we aren't always fully aware of the guilt within us, or even of the fear it arouses, we still try to get rid of it. This is a natural enough reaction, of course, though it is highly destructive. The impulse to purge ourselves of guilt is constant, demanding, and persuasive beyond estimation. It is, in essence, an instinctual psychological drive.

Perhaps the next logical questions have already occurred to you: How do we attempt to free ourselves of guilt? What is the means we use to try to purify our core? To which the answer is very simple: since we are already focused on the external world, we try to get rid of guilt by projecting it outside of us.

Now I am going to reveal something to you that is one of the universe's great keys for finding emotional balance. It is a lesson so powerful that I recommend you read it over and over until you have it memorized. Remind yourself of this lesson every morning before you start each day, and, most important, compare your experiences with it so that you can see for yourself the truth of it. It is this: anger, in any form, is nothing more than the attempt to project our own sense of guilt onto someone else in order to see ourselves as relatively innocent by comparison. When you are angry, you want another person to suffer, to feel bad for what they've done, so that your own guilt appears to be lessened. Nobody who is angry wants the problem solved. What they want is for the other person to admit their guilt. We've all experienced this from both sides.

Internalized guilt leads to fear, which in turn leads to guilt's projection — anger. This cycle plays out in our world in many ways. Have you ever noticed that when one person attacks another, the attacker often tries to blame the victim for it? A woman cheats on her husband and gets caught, and suddenly it's *his* fault. If he had been more attentive to her needs, she never would have cheated. Of course! Or a rapist assaults a woman and tries to blame her for his crime. She was *asking for it*, after all, wearing a short skirt and flirting with him. And everyone knows how politicians love to point fingers at each other when their policies fail. These are just a few choice examples of an endless game of pin the blame on the donkey, the donkey being whoever happens to be most convenient at the time. This game has millions of variations, because we live in a world of endless forms. Look at your own life in honesty and you will see many examples of it. Everyone is sick with this vicious cycle to one degree or another. It is the great disease of our species.

The interesting thing is, the anger we use to try to expel guilt never works. If it did, there wouldn't be a problem for long. You would get angry and then you would feel better. *Problem solved!* But that's not how anger operates. In fact, anger serves only to reinforce guilt, because afterward you feel doubly guilty for attacking.

Let's go through this one more time: Guilt leads to fear, which in turn leads to guilt's projection — anger. The anger then strengthens the guilt, feeding energy back into the cycle. This endless, self-sustaining loop is the mechanism that locks us into a focus on the external world, turned away from our core self, which we believe is poisoned with guilt.

Have you ever wondered why human beings are so quick to attack each other? Have you ever wondered where your own impulses to attack come from? Perhaps in most cases you justify your behavior in the name of "defense," but if you are like most people, you have experienced many powerful attack impulses that you could not fully justify or explain. The guilt cycle is the fuel behind these urges, whether or not you find a way to rationalize your feelings and behavior. This is nothing to feel additionally guilty about. Everyone suffers from this same disease. We are looking at it now only so that we might find a way to heal it.

Now, perhaps you believe this, perhaps you don't. I merely present it here for your consideration without defense or argument. With that said, I have come to understand, through my own firsthand experience, that the key to attaining emotional balance lies in nothing more complex than breaking this cycle. As you begin to relinquish the constant urge to attack and turn your attention toward healing your own sense of guilt instead, your entire psyche balances out. Gone are the ups and downs of life, and negative emotions are gradually replaced by the mind's inherent nature, which is calm and joyful. By challenging this cycle, you can achieve the type of equanimity very few even imagine is possible. Yet it is more than possible, being the basic structure of the mind, which has been hidden — but not destroyed — beneath the layer of guilt.

Breaking this cycle is also of critical importance to deepening your meditative practice, since the guilt cycle creates such a turbulent emotional environment that it makes meditation seem far more difficult than it is. While guilt remains rooted in your mind, turning inward seems fearful. Fear may be hidden beneath other *seeming* obstacles to meditation, such as restlessness or monkey mind, but the guilt cycle lies at the heart of every obstacle. Seek only to heal this cycle, and you will have no trouble meditating.

Begin this healing process by taking a forceful stand against it, and begin behaving and thinking in a manner that represents its opposite. Attributes like unconditional love, gentleness, forgiveness, compassion, noncontrol, nonjudgment, open-mindedness, innocence, gratitude, honor, respect, and patience reduce guilt and fear. This is why Christ taught forgiveness and Buddha taught compassion.

Of course, you may not feel at first that any of these positive characteristics realistically represent who you are or who you *believe* you are. Perhaps you do not think of yourself as patient, holy, or innocent. Without a doubt, starting this new direction can be difficult at first. My advice during this beginning stage is simply to bear with it and take one step at a time. Moving in the direction of peace gets much easier as you progress and gain momentum.

At first you may feel as if you are fighting your own nature, and perhaps even being dishonest with yourself and others, but this perspective is reversed. By viewing ourselves as anything but holy, innocent beings filled with compassion, forgiveness, and unconditional love for all living creatures, we are being dishonest about who we are, because our core self is all these things and many more. When we look at ourselves in a negative light, we are therefore not seeing what we really are, but rather our own images and beliefs. And this is *always* an ego viewpoint.

As your meditations grow richer, you will fall in love with the beauty you discover within yourself. Your core self has not been damaged by guilt, fear, or attack. It is still as spotless and beautiful as it was when it was created, being a direct and perfect extension of Source. Don't allow any fear or guilt to dissuade you from your search for your true identity. All the images and experiences of this world are just passing clouds that hide your awareness of core self. The truth is still within you, and the truth is this: You are more than just a body, and nothing you have ever done in this world, and nothing others have done to you, has ever changed your core self in any way. You are Spirit, at one and at peace with all living things, past, present, and future, as they are at one with you. We are all spiritual beings having a human experience, and not the other way around. We have come to earth only to learn the art of living joyously and being at peace with those who are dear to us, ourselves, the world, and our God. We are safe. We are loved. We are Spirit. We are one.

Day 41

I rest in light. I am light.

Often, when we think of the process of *healing*, we associate it only with bodily healing. This is in keeping with the belief that the body is what we are, and all that we are. It must be obvious, though, to anyone who bothers to look closely that if healing were only about fortifying the body, the process would be useless in the long run because the body is temporary. We will discuss physical healing in more detail in the chapter "Health and Healing." The lesson for today is more fundamental and provides the theoretical basis upon which many of our ideas are built.

All healing begins in the mind, not the body. The body can be thought of as an outward reflection of our inner state; therefore, if we want to bring healing to it, we need to uncover and heal the thoughts of sickness that we hold inside our mind. It is these sickened thoughts that need healing. As the mind is fortified and made well, the body will naturally strengthen and heal in response.

The primary cause of the sickness of the mind is a lack of love, and this is only the result of the guilt cycle. Guilt is an emotional sickness, and we all suffer from it to some degree. Depression, anxiety, and all other forms of self-loathing are the results. It's rare to find anyone who has fully healed and become healthy at all levels. However, each degree of success brings us more joy and one step closer to that perfect state of health in both body and mind.

Learning to love yourself is one of the most important lessons of any spiritual path, if not the only important one. Why? Because most other lessons that you might presume to be important transfer easily from this one all-inclusive learning experience. Learn to love yourself and you will simultaneously learn to love the world, because you will, of necessity, have released your own sense of guilt. When this occurs, anger and the need to blame evaporate.

Many overlook the need to heal themselves under the false assumption that it is selfish, and, being riddled with guilt, they believe they do not deserve love. Instead, they focus their spiritual efforts primarily on the attempt to offer love to everyone else while not accepting it for themselves. As a result, they miss out on their own healing and peace of mind, and they also fail to realize the true equality of love by excluding themselves from it. Unity of life, if it is true, means that *all* of us are joined as one, and therefore we must all be equally worthy of love. Obviously, this must include you as well.

Learning to love yourself is not selfish. It is the opposite. It is a big part of reprogramming your waterfall of thought. You must learn that *all* beings are worthy of love, and so are you. When people make a mistake, when they act in hatred, they are doing so because of their own sense of self-loathing and guilt. They don't need to be judged in return. They are in pain, and they need to be healed. Recognize this powerful lesson, but don't stop with applying it to others. Transfer the lesson to yourself.

As you repeat today's thought during your meditations, try to think of yourself not as flesh and blood but as pure light energy. You are not imprisoned by your body. You can just as easily turn your attention to the realm within you, toward your real home. Trust in your inherent innocence, and not guilt. Beyond the image of your body, you are light. Beyond guilt, you are perfect.

With every thought of darkness I release,
my mind is filled with light.

When you are meditating and experience persistent feelings of anger toward a specific person or situation, or guilt about something you've done or thought, it's important to take note of these feelings. While meditation does encourage you to let such thoughts go and move beyond them, when you get stuck, it is a sign. Often, such thoughts represent unhealed areas of your life that you need to examine openly and come to peace with. This process involves, first of all, recognizing them as obstacles along your path. Don't just dismiss issues that pop up with regularity, pretending that they are not there. Calmly acknowledge them, and don't be afraid to get honest with yourself. Those who wish for peace must heal all wounds.

For instance, if someone did something to hurt you in the past, and thoughts about the incident keep presenting themselves during your meditations, instead of instantly trying to bury the thoughts in unconsciousness, follow these three steps to begin the process of healing:

1. *Recognize that your feelings about the incident or person in question are unresolved.* Therefore, they have become a scar in your mind, large or small — it doesn't matter which — and as a scar, they are blocking your meditative practice and, more generally, your peace of mind. This step simply entails becoming aware. A problem cannot be fixed until you identify it and accept it as a problem

that needs fixing. Don't be intimidated by dark feelings. They can't hurt you unless you continue to let them fester unhealed.

2. *Become determined to let them be healed.* You want happiness, peace, and enlightenment, not petty grievances. What have your grievances ever given you that turned out to be for your benefit? Consider this question well, and be fair and honest. If you discover, through your own internal inquiry, that your grievances are not as valuable as peace and healing — and you cannot have both — then you will want to set a goal to heal them. By becoming determined to heal from the outset, you are setting a positive goal, which makes it much more likely that you will succeed. (This is as true of *any* goal as it is of spiritual ones. If you want to succeed at something, start by focusing on what you *do* want instead of what you *don't* want, set positive goals, and then take one step at a time to reach them.)

3. *Finally, with the problem identified and your determination to fix it firmly in place, actively let thoughts of peace replace your inner wounds.* Kept buried in your mind, negative thoughts are the most toxic stuff of life, leading to all orders of physical and emotional dysfunctions. However, examined directly in openness and then *forgiven*, these areas of unhealed emotion can provide huge boosts to your meditative practice. With each grievance you allow to be healed, you will reap enormous rewards in terms of peace and inner joy. As you let go of darkness, light will begin filling up your mind. This is not symbolic — it is a real and active process that occurs naturally.

So how, exactly, do you replace grievances with forgiveness? You start by *practicing* with forgiveness. There is a difference between practicing forgiveness and truly forgiving. Practicing it is like dipping your foot in a pool to test the water before jumping in. In other words, you may not feel entirely successful at releasing grievances at first, but you still make the effort even if it feels half-hearted or fake in the beginning. Practice is a necessary step that precedes accomplishment. This is true of any special skill. Championship basketball teams spend most of their time in training and practice. Star musicians study for years. Scientists undergo intensive graduate schooling to prepare themselves to understand what few ever will. And those who wish to heal their mind must also prepare themselves through practice and study.

For today's practice, then, take a few minutes at the outset to examine your thoughts for any areas of unhealed trauma. Don't try to seek out every hurt or wrong you have experienced. Just make a top-three list of people or incidents that are causing you pain or that have caused you pain in the past. Then, one by one, see each as clearly as you can in your mind, and tell yourself, "This is an unhealed situation and a block to meditation." Repeat today's mantra several times, applying it to your feelings about the incident or person. Try to think of the idea for today as a healing balm while you try to sense yourself coming to peace with and letting go of all angry thoughts about the situation. Spend no more than a minute or two on each one.

After you've done this with each of your top three wounds, practice as usual, trying to let go of all thoughts and sinking deeply into your meditation. Even if you are not 100 percent successful at letting go of your anger and guilt, try to sense how even the mere attempt deepens your practice and can provide an incredible sense of relief.

Day 43

I am not my body.

This short sentence contains the whole basis for peace, the justification for forgiveness, and the direction for real hope all wrapped into one. It also describes the direction of the meditative journey and ultimately why it is a healing practice. Learning the truth behind the words "I am not my body" is a realization that occurs through experience and can never happen through study alone. Your body is an extension of what you are in truth. It is a sort of mental projection outward from core self, Spirit, and eternity into the world of time and physical space. From a bodily perspective, looking out at the external world through the body's eyes and using the body to touch, taste, and interact with the world, it becomes impossible to distinguish yourself from mere flesh and blood and bone. Only through the practice of closing your eyes, turning inward, and shutting off the bodily perspective each day for a period of time will you gradually begin to distinguish the difference between *you* and *it*.

As infants begin their journey in the world, they are not focused on their new bodies. They can't control their bodies very well because their minds are elsewhere, and they don't yet perceive the body as a prison surrounding them and locking them inside, which it eventually becomes — or *seems* to become. I say *seems* because the body cannot really contain us, and it isn't accurate to say that an infant's mind is "elsewhere." A more accurate way of describing an infant's mind is that it is *everywhere*. Infants do not perceive any boundaries containing them or shutting them off from unity with life.

Spiritual evolution involves expanding your experience of life beyond the body. We are not confined by the body to a narrow slice of time and space. Like infants, we are everywhere, a part of all lives, all people, all living creatures. We've spent many years overlearning the extremely difficult task of focusing only on what our body reveals to us through its senses. Thus, unlike an infant, we have come to think of our body as much more than just a temporary home and tool we use to interact with the outside world. We think that the body is all we are. Perhaps we "believe" in Spirit, but we no longer perceive its reality. This is how we lose our sense of connection to our core self and, by extension, our Source, which we were so identified with as young children.

During your meditations today, tell yourself often, "*I am not my body*," using this mantra as a focal point like a compass as you turn inward and seek freedom from the physical. Sense the presence of the timeless Spirit within you. We are all still children at heart, still a part of Spirit, and we can return to the full awareness that this is so through the force of our wholehearted desire combined with our daily *dharma* (spiritual commitment and practices). Each time you sit down to meditate, you are telling Spirit, "I want to remember you! I want to remember who I am! I want to remember the child in me!" These statements, which are all the same, are the most powerful declarations a person can make, because they align you with the natural inclination of the entire universe: to integrate, unite, and be one.

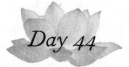

Day 44

I am not my body. I am Spirit.

So if you are not your body, what are you? This may seem a strange question, but it is the only valid question any of us can ask while self-doubt plagues us. During today's practice, as your mind begins to quiet down, remind yourself,

I am not my body. I am Spirit.

Then try to experience the truth of this statement directly. It is important to remember that although this book uses words as a part of its teaching method, words themselves can never describe our reality. Their only use is to point us in the right direction and help us to integrate peaceful thinking so that we can then experience what we are for ourselves. This experience is felt only in silence. Your own inner voice must become very quiet. Practice today listening intensely to the silence beyond your thoughts, beyond all sense of time and the physical. Reach out with your intuition and try to feel the spirit within you.

Day 45

Let me celebrate the goodness in all human beings, so that I can celebrate the goodness that resides within me.

Dr. Wayne Dyer once told a story about a tribe in South Africa called the Babemba, who have an unusual way of dealing with guilt and punishment. When one of their tribal members is accused of wrongdoing, the whole tribe stops working and gathers for a ritual trial. They take turns testifying about the accused person's past behavior. The remarkable thing is, instead of attacking the individual's past or even focusing on the present accusations, they are allowed to testify only about the person's *good* past behavior. Each tribal member comes forward and recounts, in detail, every good act and kind deed by the accused that they have witnessed. This testimony continues until everyone has had a chance to speak, a process that can go on for days. At the conclusion of the "trial," the accused is welcomed back into the tribe, and a huge celebration ensues.

Can you imagine what this does for the accused person's self-esteem? It must go through the roof! Supposedly this system is so effective at managing wrongdoing that the Babemba need to perform it only once every *four or five years*. I believe that it is so effective because they are not reinforcing guilt. Instead, they are celebrating the accused person's goodness. They are looking beyond mistakes and reinforcing positive behavior.

You can use this same tactic in your everyday life, and it is an instant life changer. You will never deal with people the same way once you see how effective this technique is for producing positive behavior and feelings. Start intentionally looking for good behavior instead of dwelling on errors, and reinforce it at every opportunity. For instance, if you have a sloppy roommate or child, instead of complaining whenever you notice a mess, offer praise when he or she has cleaned something up. Positive reinforcement is far more effective than punishment at shaping behavior because it inspires people.

Seeing the goodness in others is the opposite of judging them. You cannot see the goodness in them and judge them at the same time. Judgment always exacerbates guilt, which causes people to become defensive. This leads to a fight-or-flight response that causes them either to close off from you or to become aggressive. In contrast, seeing goodness in another has the opposite effect, and it also has one more interesting result: When you begin looking for the goodness in other people, you will begin to recognize your own inherent goodness. Through this process, you will not only inspire others and ease their sense of guilt but also inspire and heal yourself.

Day 46

Guilt is the opposite of love. I cannot experience both at the same time, and so I must choose which I want.

All negative emotions — no matter their form, their cause, or the justifications we invent to maintain them — make it impossible to love and obliterate any hope for happiness. You will know this is true if you realize that love and happiness go hand in hand and *all* negative feelings are the opposite of love. You can't experience both at the same time. You will experience one or the other at any given instant, depending on your own pervasive thinking pattern.

It often feels as though negative emotional states are imposed upon us — by other people, by external circumstances, or sometimes just by some mysterious force inside our own head that we can't pinpoint. After all, we don't actively choose fear or depression, and we justify our anger toward other people as being the result of *their* actions. We are reacting to them, and our own emotions are thus seen as more than justifiable; *they are natural.*

This is the great con by which your own emotional state is snatched from your control and placed in the hands of another or of some uncontrollable outside circumstance. If you look with clarity, you will see how allowing others to dictate your feelings deprives you of power. By letting other people determine how you feel, you are essentially throwing up your hands and surrendering to their whims, their sickness, their will. You are thus putting yourself in a position of weakness, where what *they do* and what *they say* and what *they think* have the power to dictate what *you feel*. You are giving them full authority over your most intimate assets — your mind, your feelings, your life.

Many times, it does seem as if our emotions are out of our control. Search your mind more carefully for the source of your feelings, however, and this façade begins to crumble and give way to reveal an ancient truth that is at first glance frightening, but that closer inspection reveals to be the ultimate empowerment: what needs to be healed in order for you to free yourself from negative emotions is the mother of all of them — internalized guilt. Realizing this is liberating and empowering because it gives you back control over your feelings.

We think we need to change other people to achieve happiness — to get them to behave in ways we approve of, to have them be what we want them to be. Or we think we must change the world and the circumstances of our lives. We need more money to be happy, bigger breasts, a slimmer figure. We need that promotion. We need fame, the recognition we deserve, respect and appreciation, better health, a more beautiful house, a new pair of boots, a powerboat faster than our neighbor's boat, a cabin in the mountains, more talent, more creativity, something else, anything other than what we already have, right here and right now, just as we are.

Other people may seem to be the source of our pain, and our circumstances may seem to be the cause of our dissatisfaction, but we can never find the one thing we are all seeking by changing those things outside of us. We have only one power in the world, and it is one we were born with. It is the power to choose how to view life and the world, and how to interpret the events and the people that populate our experiences here. One choice is to respond to the guilt inside you with fear and to lash out in anger in the attempt to alleviate it. The other is to look inward, challenge our own guilt, and let it be healed through the power of loving thoughts. May you choose wisely, and may today's idea help you find your way to peace. Learn to love yourself as you are, and learn to love others as they are. I urge you, look beyond mistakes of every kind and see, instead, what you are at your core. Stop responding blindly to the guilt cycle, and work to heal it instead.

Day 47

*Breathing in, my desires are one; breathing out,
my mind is at peace; breathing in, my thoughts are one;
breathing out, my mind is still.*

Another major cause of emotional distress stems from the ego's tendency to divide into different levels composed of conflicting agendas, contradictory goals, and even distinct personalities. When you have a thought system — or any system, for that matter — that contains differing objectives, conflict becomes inevitable. This is precisely the same type of clash that occurs when two people want mutually exclusive things. A husband wants to paint the house white, but his wife prefers green. Their desires conflict and a struggle of wills ensues. Even if one "wins" with relatively little conflict, the other will still feel slighted, and they are bound to be resentful, causing an imbalance in the relationship. So nobody wins.

In the same way, internal conflict occurs when you simultaneously want two or more things that are incompatible. For instance, dieters often experience this type of conflict when one part of them wants to eat a fattening meal and another part wants to lose weight. They can't have both, and so this sets one aspect of their mind at odds with another.

Many such wars are being waged in all of us — some of them major, but most relatively minor and uneventful in the grand scheme. For instance, a man loves animals and wants a dog, but he doesn't want to pay for a bigger place with a yard. A woman wants the stability of married life but is scared of commitment. A man hates his job but loves the money. A kid wants to go join his friends for a game of ball, but his favorite television show is on. A smoker wants her addiction but does not want the diseases associated with it.

Take a few minutes now to identify some of the ways your own mind is at war with itself or has been in the past. Identify the feelings these struggles have produced. Often, when we are at war on the inside, the battle finds its way into our external affairs as well. We become irritable or depressed, which can affect many things in our life, including our relationships.

The only way to free the mind from this type of internal conflict is by adopting a solitary, driving focus toward *one goal*. When you are focused on only one goal instead of many, you unify your thoughts so that they are no longer conflicting with each other, thereby eliminating the inner struggle that comes from maintaining mutually exclusive goals. Once you have only one major life goal, all the other little goals that come and go then become means of contributing to that bigger goal. If they don't help you to reach your greater goal, you simply discard them.

In my own search for peace, I have found the goal of happiness to be the most useful unifying goal. Happiness makes such a powerful and natural unifying goal because, more than anything else, basic happiness is what we all want. If you look deeply, happiness is the motivation behind *all* our separate objectives. For instance, when we are struggling with the desire to be thin versus the desire to eat a cupcake, being happy, fulfilled, and at peace is what we are really after. One aspect of our mind tells us that being thin will make us happy; the other half advises that eating the cupcake will.

Which is right? As it turns out, both are wrong. Neither being slim nor eating a cupcake will make you or me happy. Only the relinquishment of the struggle between the two warring objectives will. When a husband and wife fight over which color to paint their house, they are engaging in a conflict that is bound to add to unhappiness. Whether the house is painted white or green is meaningless in terms of producing joy. Being in a state of harmony and sharing in your partner's joy are what counts.

Integrating the levels of your mind becomes possible when you make one major but very simple change in your thinking. You have to decide with clear conviction that more than anything else in the world, more than any other objective, circumstance, or possession, you want simple happiness and peace. That's all. Nothing more, but also nothing less.

You must also understand that true, lasting happiness is an *internal state* that is not dependent on the external world in any way. If it were, happiness would be nothing more than an impossible dream, because life in the external world will always entail some difficulties. It is not stable, being a world *of change*. Lasting happiness is impossible to find while you depend on the world to produce it. However, it is equally true that once you realize happiness to be a state of mind, it is easy to achieve.

Day 48

I bless my past. I bless my future.
In the present moment, I am at peace.

Today our focus will be on thankfulness. The ego is never thankful. It focuses only on pain and stores its wounds in its own psychic body, drawing from them negative energy that it uses as food to build itself up and make itself feel more secure in pain. The ego literally feeds on negative images and thoughts. In this way, old wounds are cherished, and they will continuously poison your life in the present until they are uprooted and healed.

Becoming thankful for your life and relationships dissolves the ego. Just as seeing the goodness in others reduces guilt, thankfulness is a great healer of the guilt cycle because it eliminates the urge to attack. Use today's thought to bless all the experiences that have shaped your life and made you who you are today — even the painful ones. Try to find some little light within them that you hadn't noticed before, and focus only on that. Even the painful moments are worthy of thankfulness, because they have brought you to this moment in your life, when you have decided on a course of conscious awakening and self-exploration. In my view, pain can serve only one useful purpose: to ignite your desire to heal.

Also, try to look on the future with the awareness that everything will work out in a way that provides you with every opportunity to learn how to live a happier, more joyous life; that you will meet and pass through all difficulties safely; and that your ultimate destiny is one of eternal safety. In short, bless both your past and your future, and you will find the key to present happiness.

Day 49

Sacrifice is another form of attack upon myself.
It brings only deprivation, which, like fear,
is the opposite of love.

Plenty of meditation teachers and traditions take a hard line when it comes to "worldly pleasure seeking." This is also typical of many organized religions. From vows of celibacy to dictates about what may be consumed and when, it seems there is quite a lot of concern over what one may or may not do with one's body and still remain sanctified. Yet, curiously, each religion and each teacher seems to harbor a different view of what is acceptable in this regard. Some say you shouldn't drink alcohol, and others that you shouldn't consume even caffeine. Still other teachings advise that you should avoid having sex, or, alternatively, that you can't have sex with someone of the same gender. And on and on and on... The individual beliefs may vary, but they all share the universal theme that in order to find Paradise, you must control your behavior in one way or another.

My own advice regarding behavior is somewhat different. First, let's be clear: When we are talking about changing a person's behavior, we are talking about changing an *effect* while ignoring the *cause* of the behavior. For instance, if people want to have sex, what good is avoiding the physical act? Even if they don't act out their desires, their minds are still caught up in sexual fantasy. In fact, avoiding acting on desires can make it doubly difficult to progress beyond them, because we eliminate the opportunity to see that the things we desire are not nearly as satisfying as spiritual release. How can we tell? The idea of sex becomes a god to people who want it but refuse to act on their impulse. Their mind gets caught up in thoughts of sex, but with no hope for release. Furthermore, because they've been told that their desires are wrong, they now feel guilty about their thoughts. See how this reinforces the guilt cycle?

Trying to control your behavior without addressing the underlying thoughts is like trying to repair your car's engine by painting the car a pretty new color. It may look nicer, but you aren't going to get far in it. This sort of thinking is completely meaningless, and it leads to absolutely no advancement. On the contrary, it is likely to cause at least a minor setback along one's spiritual path. Not only does denying desires exacerbate guilt and block students from the opportunity to compare their physical, worldly impulses with spiritual experience, but it also induces a state of deprivation, and deprivation is a form of depression. Even the words are similar: *deprive*, *depress*. The true spiritual path is not a path *toward* joy. It is the path *of* joy. It is meant to add to your abundance, not take away from it.

To deprive yourself of something you are still attached to is generally not the best path. We might at times need to make big, immediate changes because a particular behavior is highly destructive to ourselves or to others. I am close to someone who is a severe alcoholic, and there is no doubt that he needs to stop drinking *now*. He is destroying his body, and his disease has already ruined many of his relationships. Most of the time, however, we are not talking about such critical issues. For the most part, the challenge of spiritual development has nothing to do with a person's behavior. Our actions derive from our thoughts. It is thought that inspires everything we do with our bodies. For us to evolve, then, it is thought that must change. Behavioral shifts will occur naturally. I am not so concerned with what my students are doing with their bodies. I am much more concerned about what is going on with their minds. One of the beautiful things about meditation is that it is a gentle path. It doesn't require you to make huge changes to your lifestyle. The major changes it asks for are changes in the way you think, view your life, and handle your relationships. Don't be tempted to walk the path of deprivation. If you want to sacrifice something, try sacrificing hatred, sadness, and all sense of self-loathing. Just take every dark feeling you've ever wrestled with, wrap it up, and throw it away forever. Give up your dedication to darkness — whatever the form — and become dedicated to happiness and peace instead. There is no worthwhile sacrifice but this, and can such an act really be called a *sacrifice*? Otherwise, changing your behavior while retaining the thinking patterns behind it will get you nowhere. All you will be doing is spinning your wheels, going nowhere in a car with a busted engine and a shiny paint job. You can't change your heart by changing your actions, but you can change your heart by changing your mind about what is important to you, what it is you value. Seek only the peace that comes from union with your core self, and all the little habits that haunt you now will naturally loosen their grip. This happens very simply when you realize that they are no longer meaningful to you. You have found something far greater, and only that can fulfill your soul now.

Thoughts are the carpenters of my life. Let me select my thoughts with wisdom, then, to reflect only the things I want to feel, for my thoughts are my gifts to myself.

The deeper you go in meditation, the closer you come to the core of your thoughts — the generator — and it is at this fundamental level that we are able to make fundamental shifts in the way we think. Since our thoughts shape our lives, reaching down into the depths of our mind places us in a position of authentic power. Now we can look at all the things within us that need healing, the hurts we have had and those we have given too, and learn to forgive both. This heals us and changes the pattern of our thoughts — and, by extension, the shape and direction of our lives.

Let me remind you, the purpose of reprogramming your waterfall is not to *do away* with your thoughts but rather to reshape them so that they bring you peace, happiness, and health instead of conflict, sorrow, and disease. Life doesn't have to be so stressful. The waterfall of thoughts you are becoming aware of through meditation runs all day, every day. Psychologists refer to these deep-set mental patterns as *scripting*. Likewise, computer specialists use the term *scripting* to describe programming language that controls various software applications. Our thoughts are much like computer scripting, in that they continuously shape our lives, even during times when we are unaware that it is happening. Going into deep meditation, into the inner mind, helps you to become aware of the nature of your thoughts, and as you work with the daily exercises in this book, you are introducing fresh new programming into your thought system. Thus you are altering your scripting directly. This is why I suggest using the focus sentences during meditation, when you are in close alignment with your core self. Doing so inserts these thoughts at a deep level. Eventually, the result is a shift in *all* the thoughts you think. Every time you think a thought of peace, especially when you are quiet and turned inward, your waterfall shifts a little more in line with core self.

Changing your scripting is the only change that will last, because by doing so, you are altering the programming of your life. Do not settle for anything less, or you will only be wasting your efforts.

The Law of Reciprocity

Giving and receiving are one and can never be separated. What you give away always comes back to you. By learning to give only what you value, you empower yourself and actively shape your life.

With today's idea, we are beginning to uncover the heart of the meditative curriculum. It is about changing not behavior but thought, and it doesn't ask for big changes but for small, gradual ones. It asks us to change our attitudes, the way we relate to others, the way we view life, and even the way we see ourselves.

Understanding the law of reciprocity is one more powerful tool for becoming a more actualized, aware human being. This ancient law, which is not a law of humankind but a natural law of the universe, has historically gone by other names, such as *karma* and *retribution*. I prefer to use the word *reciprocity*, however, for the same reasons why I prefer the word *Source* over *God*. For one thing, *reciprocity* is more descriptive and therefore can better help us to understand the phenomenon. Also, the words *karma* and *retribution* have been abused over the years by people seeking to justify their own judgments and hurtful actions.

The law of reciprocity states that giving and receiving are joined and can never be experienced independently of each other.

By choosing one, you automatically choose the other. What this means is, when you give something to someone else, even at the level of thought, you will receive whatever it is you gave. This is true because in reality, life is one, which means there is no "someone else" to give to. Let's examine this connection more deeply.

It is true that giving and receiving do not always appear to be linked. It seems that when you give something away, you lose it, but this is true only at the level of form. In form, *yes*, the things you give away may change; however, the idea — that is, what the form *represents* — is always returned. For instance, let's say you give five dollars to a homeless person. For many people, money is the ultimate representation of security in our world. In this case, what you are giving is not five dollars, which is only the form, but the idea of *security*. You have given security to another, and security, in whatever form is most meaningful to *you* based on your current circumstance, is what you will receive from the universe. Perhaps it will come in the form of money, or it could be in the form of security in your relationship, or job security, and so on. The content of the giving is what the universe registers and gives back to you. This is as true of physical "things" such as cash as it is of intangibles like acceptance or rejection, love or hatred, forgiveness or condemnation. When you give any of these things away, they also will come back to you. This law of the universe has no exceptions.

Another important point is that the law of reciprocity operates on all levels, not only physically. It is equally true of what you *think* about others. Actions are only the expressions of our thoughts, emotions, and desires. They are an effect of a cause, which originates with our thinking. Therefore, consequences are formed and given their power at the level of *thought*. Because of this, you also bring upon yourself the consequences that you only *wished* upon another.

The law of reciprocity is precisely what makes developing loving-kindness as a general attitude so effective at deepening meditation. As you begin to express only kindness in both attitude and behavior, you see these same feelings returned to you, and you grow increasingly peaceful and intolerant of conflict.

At first it may be difficult to see that your thoughts have an immediate and direct effect on you. This is not always easy to perceive, but let's take an example and observe how this works in a way that may be easier to understand. When you are angry with another person — and I mean *really* angry — isn't it true that it is *you* who suffers? Consider what happens when you are in such a state. Your mind fills with turmoil and hatred. Perhaps you even seek to defend yourself in your imagination or out loud to other people — it doesn't matter which — listing and sub-listing all the many ways the other person attacked you and how you didn't deserve it. Sometimes our anger can be so intense that it stays with us for days at a time, invading even our sleep with nightmares. This is a deeply depressing and exhausting way to live. When you're stuck in such a state, nothing seems right or good. Negative thoughts always lead to negative feelings.

Virtually everyone has experienced this type of reaction to one degree or another, and there is no cause for it beyond our own thoughts and interpretations of another person's actions. We may blame someone else for our pain, but it's primarily our own thinking process that does the most damage. This is a trick of the mind that blinds us to the truth that giving and receiving are the same. We think our feelings come from other people's actions, but it is our own *reactions* that torture us.

And what about when you are only a "little angry" with another person? Well, then you will suffer a "little pain" in return. But a lack of peace is a lack of peace. There is no joy in it.

At some point, everyone needs to recognize that the pattern of attack/defense/counterattack is endless in this world. It ends only when you become determined to take responsibility for your own feelings and actively begin managing your mind. This is the mark of emotional maturity.

Learning the secret of the law of reciprocity places you in a position of tremendous power. Very few realize this ancient truth, but it is the key to taking charge of your life and emotions, and to finding both peace and prosperity. Once you have come to realize through the fullness of your own personal experiences that thinking negative thoughts leads directly to pain, while thinking positive ones brings joy, your entire viewpoint changes. From your new perspective, when others attack you, you will realize that they are only following their own negative thinking patterns and, in so doing, are unknowingly binding themselves to this disastrous cycle. They need to learn this lesson just as much as you do.

So here is the secret to peace in this world, stated in plain words you can use every day to bring yourself the miracle of happiness: As thoughts of war lead to war, so do thoughts of peace lead to peace. If it is joy you want, offer joy to others — even in your thoughts. In fact, whatever it is you want out of life, learn to give it to other people. Begin guarding your thoughts with the vigilance of a watchdog, remembering that your mind — being an earthly extension of Source — is the most precious thing in the world, and also the most powerful. Thoughts are pure creative forces, and they always have consequences, which are either pleasant or unpleasant, depending on their nature.

Begin today to think of your mind as a holy temple, and do not allow the stillness of this temple's walls to be disturbed by unworthy thoughts — and any thought that does not reflect unity, joy, and peace *is* unworthy. Instead, let all your thoughts be purified and replaced by their peaceful opposites. Then you will see how balanced your emotional landscape can be, how many riches you already possess, and how beautiful your relationships can become. Such is the power of learning that giving and receiving are one.

Day 51

I cannot change the law of reciprocity.
My only power lies in deciding what I receive
by deciding what I give.

At first, you may experience some resistance to accepting the idea that giving and receiving are directly connected. This resistance does not stem from disbelief, however. Disbelief may be an initial reaction, but the law of reciprocity is not difficult to see in action, once you start paying attention. Give it a fair and honest try, and you will see that it works. Rather, the resistance stems from the ego's need for the continuance of negative emotions, which are its primary energy source. Negative emotions keep you feeling separated from others, which in the simplest terms is exactly what ego is: *the idea of separation*. It does not want you to know that the law of reciprocity is real, because if you do, you will realize that you can be free from negative feelings. Therefore, it must convince you that you are powerless to control your own state of mind. Keeping you focused on external problems and conflict is its primary way of doing this.

The law of reciprocity is threatening to the ego precisely because it is so predictable and easy to see. As you practice watching your thoughts and the feelings they produce, you will begin to make the connection that negative thoughts bring you pain, while positive thoughts bring you peace. It's a simple cause-and-effect relationship that is difficult to overlook once you know it's there.

Learning to fully embrace the law of reciprocity and use it to your full advantage is a different matter. Even after you realize its truth, it takes time and practice to master, mainly because we have

151

been locked into our ego's thought system for most of our lives. Mastering it doesn't need to take long at all. The law of reciprocity is in full effect in your life right now, and you can use it to come to peace immediately.

Practice watching the effects of your thoughts, beginning today. As has often been suggested, use today's idea during your meditations and also as you interact with others throughout the day. Pay careful attention to your thoughts and feelings, and take note of their connection and relationship to your experience: when you project happy, peace-filled thoughts toward others, you feel happy and at peace; likewise, when you think negatively about another person, no matter the justification, you feel pain. The more deeply you realize this truth, the faster you will progress toward reprogramming your thought system and freeing yourself from the guilt cycle.

Day 52

*Today I will learn to respect my mind,
and I will guard my thoughts with loving tenderness.*

Since your thoughts fill your mind from the instant you wake to the time you fall asleep, choosing your thoughts carefully is wise. They are your most intimate company in life; your guide through the world; your interpreter of everything you see, hear, and experience. Think about that for a moment. Every human companion in your life will come and go, but your thoughts will be with you from birth to death, during every instant. Their impact is inestimable. They dictate how to feel about yourself, your life circumstances, your relationships. They have a direct impact on whether you succeed or fail; experience health or illness, depression or joy; and on and on and on...

Learn to guard your mind with tender care and tenacity, and do not allow negative thoughts about anyone, including yourself, to abide there unchallenged. Above all else, respect your mind, respect your thoughts, and respect the minds and thoughts of other people. There is no faster or more effective way to change your life than by changing your thoughts. This change can be felt instantly. Begin by reprogramming your inner voice with today's central thought. Make it a part of your life by repeating it often and reflecting on it whenever you have even a minute of free time. In this way, you will give it a space in your thoughts and make it a part of your mind, a permanent thought.

Day 53

Anger cannot put out the light that shines within me,
but it can eclipse the light's full radiance.

A nger's real effect is to obscure, not to destroy. Anger creates a thick fog within us that temporarily envelops the core self, hiding it from our sight. Yet core self is still present, and it remains strong in its original condition — unperturbed, unchallenged, and unchanged. Its light is not extinguished because of our anger, and it is not wounded in any way by either our actions or our inattention to it. Blindness can take away only our ability to see. It has no power to change what is there, within us.

Today we celebrate the fact that our original self has not been defiled by our mistakes, our anger, or our guilt. No matter what errors we have made, no matter how great our fury has been in the past, no matter how many times we have given in to the impulse to attack, we are still free to reunite with our core self and be free of the sting of rage and the bitterness of guilt. Anger may seem powerful, but it exists only near the surface of the mind, and as you let it go, its effects dissipate rapidly. Beneath all the chaos you may have experienced in your life, your core self remains safely within you, in its original, pure, innocent state. Match its state of purity by purifying your thoughts. By doing so, you will alleviate the fear of guilt that keeps anger alive; and as anger goes, you will see that nothing you have ever done, said, or thought has wounded your core. It is still safe within you. It is still at peace. It is still perfect. And it is still your true home.

Day 54

When I am kind and merciful to the world,
it is kind and merciful to me.

Many people suffer from a tendency to see themselves as victimized by the world. The victim role is related to the ego's need to make us feel powerless. Many meditation students go through a stage during which they believe that becoming a gentle person means they should allow other people to abuse them. However, the victim role is nothing more than the reverse of the aggressor role, and neither reflects the strength of Spirit. They are flip sides of the two primary ego characteristics. Look more carefully at the role of victim, and you will realize that it is a position of weakness. It testifies to the idea that life can be attacked and that you are frail and vulnerable.

The true spiritualist, on the other hand, sees that only the physical body can be injured and only the conditions of the ego are subject to decline, whether through natural atrophy or intentional assault. Our core self is a direct extension of Spirit, whose strength and power are without limits. To view yourself as a victim is to view yourself as a body and an ego. Flip your perspective around, and you will understand that what you are in truth cannot be assailed, threatened, or damaged in any way.

A very real and dependable strength comes from embracing gentleness grounded in the realization that you are infinite and all-powerful. This realization brings openness and clarity, as well as a nondefensiveness that can come only from knowing that you are absolutely safe, now and forever. You cannot be a victim. You cannot be taken advantage of. You cannot be attacked.

By choosing gentleness, you are choosing to love yourself, and as you do so, being either a victim or an aggressor will lose its appeal. There is no weakness in becoming a warrior of peace. Unless they are trying to teach a specific spiritual lesson, the gentle do not allow themselves to be abused.

Just as you should be vigilant against thoughts of attack toward others, you should be equally alert to feelings of victimization. Become strong and grounded in your spiritual reality, and learn to see compassion and gentleness as strengths, not weaknesses. Then you will come to understand that you deserve mercy, like all the world, and you won't be inclined to either abuse or be abused.

Day 55

*Because giving is receiving,
every form of healing must come from my own
willingness to extend thoughts of healing to others.*

Instead of focusing on actions, meditation teaches you the importance of acknowledging and respecting the power of thought. All actions, and in fact all things physical — whether positive or negative — originate at the level of thought. *Intention*, the great engine behind everything we experience on the physical plane, exists inside the mind; therefore, to change the things outside you, you first have to change the things inside you. Likewise, to heal the body, it is necessary to change the thoughts that contribute to its diseases. When you extend thoughts of peace and wellness to others, thoughts of peace and wellness will return to you. The body cannot help but respond.

We have already said that whatever the circumstances you wish to heal or change, whether physical, emotional, or circumstantial, you must begin by focusing on changing your thinking pattern. One way to begin this process is by setting your intention each morning to live a conscious life, which essentially means becoming aware of your thoughts and how they shape your experiences. This was discussed in an earlier section of the book, but it is such a powerful practice that it deserves repeating. If there are changes you would like to see happen, start your day by visualizing those changes during your morning meditation, and try to feel as if they are already a reality. Hold them in your mind as clearly as you can, and trust this exercise to transform your intentions into reality. Visualizing your intentions as specifically as you can is a powerful exercise.

This procedure doesn't need to last more than a minute, and, to reiterate, your morning meditation is the perfect opportunity to set your objectives for the day ahead. By doing this regularly, you will begin to see how you can live a life of conscious intention instead of a life controlled by the unpredictable actions of the world outside.

Day 56

*I extend thoughts of peace and well-being
to everyone I meet or think of today,
that I may abide in everlasting peace along with them.*

Our thoughts unite on a collective level to shape the planetary conditions of the earth. Most people never even suspect this. Even those who have learned that their thoughts are the master craftsmen of their own lives often miss this related point. As you learn to dive more deeply into your core, you will begin to realize that you do not exist in a state of isolation from other people. Just beyond the appearance of separateness, we are all linked together in the body of Spirit. Don't take this as mere spiritual speculation, for it is a phenomenon you can experience directly, given the proper training and, most important, desire. Your personal thoughts reach inward into the collective consciousness of our entire species, and as they do so, they join with other thoughts, positive or negative, depending on your state of mind. Masses of negative thinking patterns create negative circumstances on earth, and positive thoughts unite with other positive thoughts, shaping our planetary conditions in constructive directions.

This is another reason why meditation cannot be considered a selfish act. As you change the direction of your thinking, you join the worldwide effort with many other teachers of peace to shift the direction of the entire planet toward healing. This can hardly be considered anything other than the most profound mission of all sentient beings. To join in the collective effort to heal our planet by repairing it at its most fundamental level is certainly a calling worth taking part in, if ever there was one.

I invite you to remind yourself how profound your thoughts

are and how they influence a range of life far greater than anything your eyes can detect. They have an influence on everyone you see and think of, and everyone who sees and thinks of you, for we are all joined together in a union that extends forever. Imagine life as a great ocean in which we all live. The conditions of that ocean affect us all. Don't poison our home with negative energy. You can just as easily lighten up and offer peace instead. In fact, aligning with peace is easier because there is no strain involved. You have the power to make this shift. Your thoughts affect far more than just you. What begins as one thought of peace, one wish for happiness, one call for unity, will grow with love into a mighty force for global change. As you give, you receive. The law of reciprocity has no limits. You may extend peace to others through your actions, your thoughts, or your words, and you may do so at the individual or collective level.

Day 57

*Depression obliterates joy from my awareness,
but joy, like my core self, can never be destroyed.
It is as eternal as the Source of joy itself.*

Can joy be hard to experience? In our world, it does often seem that way. Yet the law of reciprocity can be used as a tool to make this transition easier, and the change need not take long. You can change your thinking pattern instantly. Just as depression obliterates joy from your mind, so too does joy obliterate depression. This is why the shift from depressed thinking to joyful thinking can happen so rapidly. Joyful thinking is strange and not understandable from a mind-set dominated by negative energy, but the reverse is true as well. Thoughts of joy are ruinous to thoughts of pain. As you begin thinking joyful thoughts, even if you are not fully committed to this new way of thinking at first, your early attempts will help depression to dissipate.

Why is it so easy? Joy is the natural condition of your mind, and therefore negative thinking patterns cannot damage or destroy it. Depression, fear, and attack exist only on the surface of the mind. Underneath every negative feeling you experience, joy fills your mind. Picture the ocean. Storms may rage at its surface, winds howl, swells rise, and waves break and crash, but the depths of the sea are completely unaffected. So it is with your mind. The mind's inherent joy can be temporary eclipsed by dark feelings while you remain on its surface, but that doesn't mean the joy is gone. Your mind is made of joy. Joy *is* the ocean. Just change your thinking by ever so little, investing each day in peace, and the natural joy that is everywhere will bubble to the surface of your life. You cannot feel this joy while storms of anger rage in your mind; however, that does not mean the joy is not there. Use the law of reciprocity to master the art of joyful thinking and become free of depression.

Day 58

I rest in gentleness.

Think of meditation as rest, not work. It is sacred time you set aside each day to step back from the world and all the busyness and stress of daily life, and to sink into quietness for a little while. This does not involve strain. If it helps, imagine that meditation is like your own personal day spa in which you allow yourself to relax and be at peace for a change. This is why meditation is so healing. The world wears us down with constant stress, while meditation reconnects us to the inner state of peace, where we destress, unwind, and rebalance in the ultimate sense of the word. Meditation is a massage for your mind and soul.

"I rest in gentleness, I rest in gentleness, I rest in gentleness." Let this message fill your consciousness as you meditate today. Think nothing else, hear nothing else, and feel nothing else. Come away from today's practicing rejuvenated, quiet in heart, and more serene.

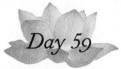

Day 59

May the peace of meditation extend through me,
surrounding and protecting me all through the day.

It isn't necessary to limit the peace of meditation to your formal practice times. Try to feel peace extending from your meditations to abide with you even as you go about your ordinary business of the day. We mentioned this already, but today we will reinforce this point. Many students limit peace to the periods of time they set aside for formal meditation. Once their practice is over, they quickly dump the peace they've accumulated and go back to business as usual. What a waste! Meditation can help you in more ways than just your formal practicing. Why limit peace? Doing so will greatly slow your progress, not only by restricting the peace you could experience all day long but also by interfering with your next meditation period. If you allow your mind to slip away from the meditative experience, the next time you sit down to practice will be doubly difficult because you'll be spending most of your time just trying to get settled and unwind.

Fill up on peace during your morning practicing; and when you are done, try to keep your mind focused on the feeling of being centered and balanced, quiet and still, light and free, that meditation fosters. Attempt to bring these feelings with you as you move ahead with your day, so that you will remain anchored to this state. You will see what a difference it makes in terms of easing stress and inspiring joy — not only in you, but in everyone you come in contact with.

Also, by remembering your focus sentences periodically during the day and taking a moment or two to reconnect with inner stillness, you will help keep your mind in a more balanced state. This will enhance your meditations and also guard your thoughts all day long. Aim to remember the daily thought at least several times each day — or, better yet, try to think of it every hour. You need to take only enough time to repeat it once or twice, thoughtfully, until you feel it engaging your attention and bringing you a sense of tranquillity. If you have time for it, you will also certainly benefit from taking a minute or two to close your eyes and do a short meditation sometime in the midday.

Day 60

Just as thoughts of peace return peace to me, thoughts of prosperity bring prosperity, thoughts of abundance give abundance, and thoughts of health produce wellness.

One final point regarding the law of reciprocity is that it is unbiased and unlimited. Once again, it is a simple cause-and-effect law that doesn't judge what you should have or be deprived of. It doesn't know the difference between good and evil, wealth and poverty, joy and sadness, health and sickness, or abundance and lack any more than a computer program would. *Your thoughts create.* That's the rule. Therefore, you can use the law of reciprocity to bring you all the things you value and simultaneously reduce the things you don't wish to experience.

Just be certain you are paying attention to the content of your thoughts and not just their form. For instance, often a concern about money leads to thoughts of impoverishment, although on the surface you may be attempting to think in line with abundance. True abundance thoughts, however, reflect the notion that you have all the money you need to get you through the day, coupled with the faith that should any unforeseen needs arise today or tomorrow, the universe will provide. Your needs will be met because we live in a universe that gives and gives without restraint or judgment. The presence of fear — or any level of concern, for that matter — is an indication that you are not in line with abundance.

Once more, the law of reciprocity registers only the *content* of your thoughts. This needs to be fully understood, but it's not an entirely alien notion. It is similar to how we judge other people in everyday life. Imagine, for instance, your significant other coming home one day from work, clearly angry. They slam the door, head to the kitchen, and start banging around, opening and slamming cabinets, and so on. You can tell they are angry, but when you go in and ask them what's wrong, they turn and shout, "Nothing!" Would you believe that nothing was wrong? Of course not. You would see beyond their words, judging their actions. You are no fool, and neither is the universe. To change your thoughts to reflect the things you want, you must reach deep down inside and change their essence.

The *Real* Justification for Forgiveness

In the world of separation, we believe that we are walled off from one another by our bodies and must seek to protect this state through our attitudes, judgments, and attacks, which reinforce our sense of being different from other people. The only way to heal this condition is to lay aside all attacks and refuse to engage.

Let's face it, people hate to forgive. Some people even hate the word *forgive*. We like our grievances, and we want others to feel guilty about the hurtful things they have done to us. In fact, we like our grievances so much that we often get angry over the pettiest matters or about things that do not affect us at all. Even very spiritual people sometimes feel dishonest by attempting to forgive grievances, as if they are fooling only themselves.

This sounds horrible, of course, and even admitting to it kindles feelings of guilt. However, all healing must start with honesty, even if it causes us some temporary discomfort. We have to become willing to admit that our darkest thoughts exist before we can even consider letting them go.

You may have heard that forgiveness is a powerful spiritual tool, and indeed it is. No single practice is more effective than forgiveness at stimulating spiritual development, bringing peace of mind, and even alleviating sickness, whether of the mind or of the body. The real question is not forgiveness's value, but whether or not it is justified. Everyone must eventually ask this question.

So what is the real justification for forgiveness? To understand this, we need to first ask ourselves, What is the justification for the opposite of forgiveness — judgment and punishment? Why do we want people to feel guilty? Wouldn't it be more helpful to look at their attacks as indications that they are sick and therefore need help? Not only is this a more mature viewpoint, but also it is infinitely more helpful because it puts us in a position where healing them becomes our primary focus. When we focus on punishing others for their mistakes, it is impossible to help them. Who would accept "help" that is contaminated with judgment? Nobody wants to feel guilty. If you attack someone for their mistakes, in all likelihood you are acting from the ego, and there will be a predictable response: either they will become defensive and emotionally shut themselves off from you, or they will become aggressive and attack you in return.

People attack and do horrible things to themselves and others because they are in pain and are frightened. They feel empty, deprived, desperate. They hate themselves. There is absolutely no other cause for attack. Even when someone is trying to wrest some worldly possession or power through attack, this is still an act rooted in thoughts of separation, which is always a fear-based state. Without the belief in separation, it becomes apparent that when we attack and deprive others, we ultimately attack and deprive ourselves. As the law of reciprocity would predict, there can be no gain through conquering and depriving another.

True spiritual warriors never let their vision stop at the level of behavior. They look beyond actions and words, and straight into another's soul. If you hope to be at peace, you must learn to view attack in a new light. When people act out in anger, they are really telling us that they are in terrible pain, and they are begging for help. The bigger the attack, the louder the cry. Behind every attack — in every form — lies a wounded animal that believes it is nothing more than a speck of decaying dust without a purpose in all the great universe. Now ask yourself, if you saw that this was true, would people's attacks be forgivable or not? If you found a puppy that had been run down by a car, would you be angry if it lashed out and bit you when you tried to help it, or would you understand that its reaction was one of self-preservation? Look carefully. These questions are identical.

Let's examine the phenomenon of judgment honestly and without fear. We want others to feel guilty because it makes us feel better than them and thus alleviates a little bit of our own underlying guilt and sense of inadequacy. Feelings of superiority also cause us to feel different from them, which reinforces the belief that we are all separate from one another. Ego is strengthened by emphasizing differences.

Once you understand this, you will also understand that the fact of unity is the *real* justification for forgiveness. Why should you forgive another? When you forgive another, you are really only forgiving your own guilt. This is why forgiveness always brings *you* peace when you offer it to someone else, even when it is given in the form of a silent blessing. Do you want peace? Ask yourself this to determine if forgiveness is justifiable in your own mind, for all forgiveness is self-forgiveness. It can bring only joy to all parties involved.

Everyone has been attacked by others, in one way or another. These attacks may be physical, but more often than not, they take place in subtler ways, such as verbally or through passive-aggressive behavior. Either way, the feeling is similar. It seems to us, at least on the surface, that it is natural and justified to attack others in return, or at least to think about doing so. Yet what if you truly realized that by attacking another, you were attacking yourself? Not indirectly or metaphorically, but directly, literally. You will learn to forgive only when you learn that this is true and also that you deserve better than this. Here is another question for you: Do you think you deserve peace? For to accept it, you must realize that it is both possible *and desirable*, which means you must judge yourself worthy of receiving it.

Are you worthy of peace? Do you honestly think you deserve to be happy? Or is there some part of you that resists this and feels that you are not good enough, not strong enough, not worthy enough? Do you love yourself? Once again, consider these questions with care. Beneath their forms, they are all asking the same thing.

Here is a simple way of understanding how peace and forgiveness go hand in hand: you cannot be happy while anger is in your mind. This is a fact, and, like it or not, you will never be able to change it. If you want to be happy, you will have to forgive your grievances, both old and new.

With this in mind, you should not see forgiveness as a loss. You do not lose anything at all by forgiving another person. Your grievances have never given you anything other than pain. You don't have to take my word for this. Select any grievance you have held, old or new, and look carefully at its effects. Did it do anything positive for you or anyone else? Did it heal the situation and bring peace? Did it make you smile, filling your heart with joy and your mind with light? Forgiveness will bring you the joy of releasing the heaviness of judgment, which is far more painful than most realize. Forgiveness heals and infuses your thoughts with tranquillity and well-being. To learn to forgive, all you need to do is clearly identify the effects of both forgiveness and judgment, and decide that you want the gifts that forgiveness offers. Make this decision consciously, and set your intention to free yourself from judgment. You can do this today, and I encourage you to do so. Join with me and with many others who have begun to accept a new way of living in this world that inspires hope and focuses on healing. There are only two paths in this world, two ways of living. Judgment is one path; forgiveness is the other. Which do you prefer? The decision is yours.

Day 61

As I see others, I will see myself.

Today's idea summarizes everything we have covered recently. As you see others, you will see yourself. This is how the law of reciprocity applies to both judgment and forgiveness. By viewing other people as angry, cynical, deprived, limited, stupid, or in any way unworthy, you reinforce these characteristics in yourself. Even if the form of negativity varies, the underlying sentiment will always be translated accurately by the universe. However, it is equally true that when you choose to see others as loving, worthy, peaceful, creative, and powerful, you will begin to see yourself in these ways too. Becoming highly selective in the way you see others, then, is your ticket to empowering yourself and shaping your life in ways you may never have imagined. In fact, as this kind of thinking matures, anything becomes possible.

Today, watch your thoughts for signs of judgment about others or yourself. Whenever you catch yourself judging, make an effort to take just a moment to recall today's thought, which will remind you that you are shaping how you feel about yourself with every thought. Then switch things around. Even if you have to force yourself, take whatever judgment you've made, and replace it with an opposite thought. For instance, if you catch yourself looking in the mirror and thinking something like "I hate my crooked nose!" stop and challenge that thought. Look again, and this time tell yourself, "On second thought, I *love* my crooked nose. It's one of a kind! Nobody has a nose like mine." Simple example, right? But you get the picture. It is time to take control of your life by taking charge of your thoughts, and today's idea is an exercise in doing just that. Make this exercise a daily habit, and your days will be filled with magical discoveries about yourself and everyone who is a part of your life. You will discover just how closed off and limiting judgment is, and just how liberating choosing positive interpretations can be.

Day 62

True forgiveness and false forgiveness are opposites in every way. True forgiveness brings only release to everyone, while false forgiveness is just another form of attack.

Almost every student who is learning to practice forgiveness goes through a stage of false forgiveness. This stage of development can become seriously protracted unless a clear distinction between authentic and false forgiveness is drawn. Most of what masquerades as forgiveness is not forgiveness at all but some form of judgment. As in all things, the content behind the act of forgiveness is what makes it true or false. True forgiveness arouses feelings of release, while its false counterpart actually increases conflict by causing you to feel not only attacked but also resentful and unfairly victimized. Thus you are not released from pain and conflict but doubly imprisoned.

Because the two versions of forgiveness bring diametrically opposed results, it is essential that you learn how to tell the difference between them. True forgiveness always entails a shift away from ego, attack, and guilt. In this sense, true forgiveness can be considered an experience more than an action. It is something you feel. When you release people from your judgment at this deepest level, you acknowledge their inherent holiness despite their behavior. You experience this level of forgiveness as a lightening of pain in your own perception and a simultaneous opening to inner joy. Therefore, forgiveness is a gift you give *and* receive simultaneously.

True forgiveness does not look down on another — in fact,

just the opposite. It sees other people as being worthy beyond their own perception of themselves, beyond their behavior, and beyond their body.

You can tell the difference between true and false forgiveness simply by examining your own feelings. As long as you feel angry or resentful, or in any way not at peace, your offering of forgiveness is still limited. You can challenge false forgiveness by looking carefully at your motivations for judgment. What are you getting out of judgment that you are afraid forgiveness would take away? Do you feel inherently worthy, or are you using judgment to stymie some underlying sense of guilt and unworthiness within you? Whatever it is, you must believe that you are getting something from judgment, and this is what you need to challenge, recognizing that as you bind another to your judgment, you bind yourself to turmoil. You cannot judge another without judging yourself. Look with anger at the world outside you, and you will believe the world within you is sick. Yet, if you find a way to look with equanimity on everything and everyone, you will discover real peace within. Try to think of this cause-and-effect relationship every time you are tempted to judge instead of forgive, so that it becomes your automatic response to every situation.

Do not be satisfied with your attempts at forgiveness until your peace of mind runs so deep that no trivial upset can drag you from it. You needn't feel guilty when you fail at forgiveness, but don't use failure as an excuse to quit challenging yourself. Forgiveness, like meditation, is a gently unfolding path. Your main focus should remain on your own willingness to continue ahead, going ever deeper into its breathtaking ways.

Day 63

Forgiveness has no cost.
It is free, and it offers only freedom.

Our intentions, the things we believe are valuable, and the things we want will always guide us through life. So it is that while we believe that judgment brings us something of value, we will not accept the gifts of forgiveness. In fact, we will be scared of forgiveness, because we will believe that it robs us of our grievances. From this point of view, forgiveness seems to be nothing more than a joke, and it is just this type of forgiveness that so many people mock — and rightfully so. Not only does false forgiveness fail to heal pain, but also it is dishonest, because through it you seek to fool yourself, and others, that you are no longer angry about something when in fact you are.

Anyone who has experienced the release of true forgiveness, however, knows that it is no joke, and its power to release is without question. It isn't a nice, placating gesture but instead a liberating experience of beauty and empowerment. True forgiveness brings peace of mind, and by doing so, it aligns you with core self. Do not equate false forgiveness with true forgiveness.

Try to recognize that there is no loss in forgiveness, and also try to sense how much you stand to gain from it. Look clearly at how forgiveness's opposite — judgment — brings with it only pain, and ask yourself if the relinquishment of pain can honestly be labeled a loss. Once you are able to see the relationship between judgment and pain clearly, you will also be able to make out the correlation between forgiveness and peace. Until this becomes brilliantly clear, forgiveness is bound to remain a threatening idea, and your ability to accept it will be limited. Essentially, to embrace forgiveness, you have to realize that it gives you something you really want and value. Practice this exchange today by making every effort to extend forgiveness instead of judgment. Restrain your impulses to lash out, and learn to see others through quiet eyes that understand and look beyond mere appearances. Give forgiveness just a little space in your heart, and feel the rewards that your humble efforts can bring you.

Day 64

Compassion! Great teacher of peace!
Show me how to see with clarity,
and guide my eyes to look upon only what is true.

When others attack you, there is another way of seeing things that will help heal any situation, no matter how troubling. Over time, every attack, whether given or received, adds to our overall psychological burden, which is like a growing internal debt. Eventually this debt accrues to the point where it begins to affect our everyday functioning and ability to cope. This is why as some people age, instead of becoming wiser and more mature, they become increasingly unstable. Their own sense of personal guilt has started to overwhelm them.

Beginning today, let us stop adding to our growing internal debt of pain and turn our life-course around through our adamant decision to take things in a bold new direction. There is a better way to interpret attack that works to alleviate pain instead of adding to it. Behind every hurtful action and thought, we can allow compassion to see for us. Compassion gives you the power to look beyond the surface of all things that seem ugly and hateful, and to see the need for healing, the pleas for help, and the cries for mercy.

Deep down, everyone in the world wants peace, even when they are acting aggressively. Those who behave the most insanely are those who are twisting in the throes of humanity's greatest disease: the plague of the guilt cycle. This is the truth behind every form of attack, and the more practiced you become at spotting it, the greater your wisdom, for the eyes of compassion always see with wisdom. They don't stop at the level of petty judgments to tell them what is what. The eyes of compassion look beyond the surface and seek out the truth behind appearances.

If you manage to accomplish nothing else in your life but healing the guilt-cycle disease, you cannot help but become a teacher of wisdom. You will see life so differently that it will feel as if you have been reborn. From this newborn place of quiet and stillness within you, a space you have opened up by releasing your own sense of guilt, you will be able to see all attack as nothing more than a symptom of the same disease you have overcome. Then you will want to help others to heal when they lash out instead of being so quick to engage them on an ego level. This is the attitude that will finally make a difference in your life and will produce real changes. Within this tiny, unassuming shift in attitude, you will find a peace so rich and deep that it will drape everything you see in beauty. The eyes of compassion see beauty first in others and then invite you to turn your gaze around and look upon your own heart with purity and forgiveness. Forgive others for the things they have done to wound you, and then forgive yourself.

Let compassion show you how to do this. Just learn to be quiet and listen to its counsel. Try thinking of all people you meet as your dear brothers and your beloved sisters, who have become lost and cannot find the way to peace. Will you choose to look upon even their worst moments with mercy, or will you return attack for attack — knowing what the results will be and realizing that it is a vicious, endless cycle that goes on until it is consciously broken? Learn to love them even when they act in hatred, and you may be surprised how strongly they respond with love. As with all things, love breeds love, compassion returns compassion, and peace brings peace. Build the world you want to inhabit by investing in only the things that bring you happiness. This is the only way out of pain.

Day 65

Forgiveness is strength, and gentleness is my protector.

Many people believe, at least subconsciously, that forgiveness is a weakness. Contrary to this false perspective, forgiveness is a virtue and a strength. Only those who have accepted themselves as creations of a loving Spirit can forgive freely, because they know that what they are needs no protection. Therefore, they see no reason to defend themselves. Instead, they trust forgiveness and gentleness to protect them by shielding their thoughts from the nightmares caused by hate.

Even in obvious ways, forgiveness can be seen as a powerful asset. Those who embrace the power of forgiveness often appear to others as more emotionally mature and trustworthy. When you stop attacking others and stop engaging with people on an ego level, people begin to turn to you for help and advice. When forgiveness is your focus, you automatically shift from egotistical goals like winning or proving you are right to focusing on healing, bringing peace, and problem solving. It's a paradoxical trade-off. As you let go of ego, you begin to achieve all those things the ego is enamored of, becoming more successful on many worldly levels. Your relationships improve, growing more meaningful and fulfilling, and you develop a type of self-esteem that isn't dependent on other people's expectations and judgments of you. Think about how liberating this can be! It frees you to be yourself, and to speak and act with honesty, instead of allowing fear of what others might think about you to influence your behavior. You will also probably begin to think more clearly and become more creative, which can lead you to more financial security too.

When you compare attack-based attitudes with forgiveness, you will realize that attack — which seems on the surface to be a symbol of worldly power — is a weakness and a disability. When you are engaging in attack, other egos are drawn to attacking you back, and you will naturally feel the need defend yourself. In contrast, when you embrace forgiveness, you have a lot more reasons to relax. Attack causes you to feel paranoid and defensive. Forgiveness brings you peace and encourages health of both body and mind. Attack creates enemies. Forgiveness mends relationships and encourages others to act with kindness and compassion toward you.

Unquestionably, forgiveness is a great protector, and by clothing yourself in gentleness, you will feel more safe, loved, and cared for. There is an old Christian saying that as long as you hold Christ in your heart, no harm can come to you. The same is true of forgiveness, which is the spirit of Christ. As long as you carry forgiveness in your heart, only good can come to you.

Day 66

Emotional despair stems from judgment,
joy from forgiveness. Whenever I am unhappy, all I need
to do is forgive in order to bring my mind to peace.

Anytime you are in emotional distress, pause for a few minutes, turn quietly inward, and look carefully at what you have been thinking about during the past hours. Almost certainly, if you are able to look deeply and with honesty, you will discover that you have been harboring some unforgiving thoughts, whether about some other person or yourself.

You can choose to release negative thoughts at any given moment and instantly free yourself from their painful effects. Think of it as being like taking out the garbage. If you let your kitchen garbage sit for too long, it will begin stinking and overflowing onto the floor. Your mind is even more prone to this if you are accustomed to thinking negatively, and since your thoughts are your constant companions, you must take extra care with your mind's upkeep. When you notice things getting fouled up — a state you can easily detect by examining your emotions — pause for a minute or two to close your eyes and practice a simple exercise in forgiveness, during which you seek only to free your mind from negative thoughts and invite thoughts of harmony to replace them.

You may use any simple positive thought for this, such as today's idea, and think it over and over during a brief meditation, slowly and with careful attention, until you feel it begin to take hold and bring peace to your thoughts. Try to allow it to replace whatever negative emotions are playing in your mind. Alternatively, you can use the mantra *"peace,"* timing it with your exhalations. Once again, the specific words aren't important.

At first, you may find it difficult to break negative emotional states once they've taken root, but with determined practice you will soon become better at doing so, and the rewards are tremendous. Performed consistently, such exercise will gently show you how you can master your mind so that you rule your emotions instead of allowing them to rule you.

Day 67

My life is a reflection of all lives; my will,
a part of the Universal Will; my mind, a holy thought
of the Original Mind. When I forgive, I forgive myself.

Today our practice will be different. After you have gotten relaxed and settled into your meditation, imagine yourself sitting before a mirror. Then imagine that this mirror shows the reflection of someone you have unhealed grievances with. These grievances could be major or minor; it doesn't matter which. All unforgiving thoughts have the same effect on us. They keep us trapped in a narrow, emotionally turbulent world and encourage the growth of fear and anger, which keeps us from going deeply into meditation. For this exercise, just select the first person you can think of, and see them in the mirror, looking out at you.

Next, briefly think of your anger with them — the things that bother you most. Do not spend more than a minute doing this. You don't have to cover everything. The point of this exercise is not to dwell on your hurt feelings but to attempt to let them go. Even if you are a little successful at this, your spiritual growth will be ample.

As you look at this person, tell them, "When I forgive you, I will forgive myself. And when I forgive myself, I will be free to see myself."

Next, look carefully at the person's face, and especially at their eyes. Look for a subtle glow of light there, the spark of life we all share. See if you can find it in their face, hiding beneath their ego, which is just a façade, a mask they wear and not their true self at all. Let compassion show you how all of this person's anger, their attitude, and their hurtful actions stem from their own pain. See if you can find that truth.

Finally, try to see yourself in this person's face. Look for the similarities between the two of you — physically, emotionally, intellectually, spiritually, and so on. Most important, try to imagine their face gently morphing so that it is no longer someone else you are looking at but yourself.

Repeat today's focus sentences several times during this exercise, and then again at the end, while you are trying to uncover light within this person and sense your mutual connection. This whole exercise should not take longer than five minutes.

Finish your meditation by sitting silently in the peace that forgiveness has helped you to uncover.

Day 68

Depression is a self-attack.
I choose to forgive and bless myself instead.

There are many kinds of illnesses in the world. Some are physical, of course, but sicknesses of the mind can be just as destructive and painful as any physical disease. Depression is one of the most common of these, and it needs to be taken seriously. Most people struggle with depression to one degree or another at some point, and for many it can become debilitating. If you believe you are suffering from depression, talk with your doctor or a qualified therapist. For some, medications can be helpful, at least temporarily. Even at moderate levels, depression can sap our energy and cloud our thinking with dread, a sense of meaninglessness, and a feeling of disconnection from other people.

Beyond drugs, regular meditation is a particularly effective remedy for the symptoms of depression. Meditation works in several ways. First, it alleviates feelings of meaninglessness, one of depression's primary symptoms. On a side note, while many psychologists consider feelings of meaninglessness to be a symptom of depression, they are often a cause. This is true because, quite simply, the feeling that life is meaningless *is depressing*. In fact, all the major symptoms of depression, which also include isolation, enervation, and — in severe cases — thoughts of suicide, add to the disease, transcending their role as mere symptom. Yes, depression may cause some of these feelings, but the symptoms in turn make the depression worse.

When you connect with your core self through meditation, you infuse your life with new energy and a sense of meaning that transcends any that can be found in worldly possessions, hopes, and aspirations. When we try to rely on physical things and on worldly goals, status, and values to satisfy us, we are always disappointed in the long run. They simply do not have the power to satisfy, so if you believe that this is all you have in life, of course you are going to be depressed about it. Not only do the things of the world fail to satisfy, but also they are temporary, and even if you happen to find some worldly thing or condition that *seems* to gratify you, it is guaranteed not to last. The world itself is only temporary.

Meditation does even more than bring a sense of lasting satisfaction, however. It also increases your feelings of connection to other people, one of the primary ways of defeating depression. In one sense, depression finds its roots in a sense of isolation. Feeling alone and isolated increases our sense of meaninglessness, because life, at its purest level, is a state of absolute unity. Depression, on the other hand, is a closing down from life, a shutting off from relationships, and a loss of the realization that our lives are inherently meaningful independent of external gratifications.

The best defense against depression in the long term is to make a regular habit of meditating, preferably twice per day. By releasing your focus on the world outside you and all thoughts of external goals and situations, you will free yourself to connect with the far richer and more satisfying state of your inner world. You will also begin to build a reservoir of inner peace as your waterfall of thought changes over from ego-dominant thoughts of guilt, fear, and anger to thoughts of forgiveness, compassion, and acceptance. This transfer alone is enough to fortify your resistance to depression. With any form of sickness of the mind, it should be obvious that changing your thoughts has to be an essential element of the healing process.

If you suffer from depression, take heart. You are not alone, and there are answers. Still, it is your responsibility to make the changes that will help you to heal. As they say, the doctor can only write the prescription; it is the patient's responsibility to fill it.

Depression is one of the most common human afflictions. Don't hesitate to get help from health care professionals if you need it, but don't accept pills as a long-term cure. Such traditional treatments are not comprehensive, because medications don't change the thinking patterns that are the underlying cause of depression. While recent research indicates that some forms of depression are linked to imbalances in brain chemistry, I believe that the biochemical reactions in the brain are *effects* of the disease, not causal agents. This is why very few patients achieve lasting relief from depression through medications. Inevitably, their depression returns, or the disease shifts form to some other affliction — a phenomenon that physicians and psychologists refer to as "transfer of symptoms." Pills may temporarily help mitigate the symptoms, which is useful for giving people an initial boost out of the darkness so that they can become functional again. From there, however, patients who hope for long-term recovery need to use this fresh energy to turn their efforts toward finding and healing the root cause of their illness. Don't settle for anything less.

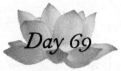

Day 69

I am safe. I am at peace. And my peace brings me joy.

Today's mantra is an affirmation that reflects a relationship not many people recognize. Peace is not a vacant, passive state that merely comes with a lack of external conflict. Real peace precipitates real joy. It is a state of empowerment, and the feelings that flow from peace can be intense. The deeper you immerse yourself in peace, the more intense the joy you will experience. One way to tell if you are experiencing real inner peace or just a passive lull in external conflict is to ask yourself, "Do I feel an inner sense of intense, unfolding joy? A sense of lightness? An active drive to forgive?" If not, you still have work to do, but don't let that upset you. You are now making the effort to heal. Be determined not to give up, and your path will only grow easier and gentler as you continue ahead.

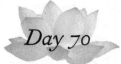

Day 70

*Spirit speaks to me through everything I see
and everyone I meet.*

The Great Spirit is not silent but speaks to us all the time,
through many channels. Spirit's language is different, however, so to hear it, you must learn to listen in a different way.

When you set aside your grievances, you open your eyes
and ears to visions that exceed worldly sights and sounds. As the
racket of our fear-based thoughts recedes, the subtler sounds of
Spirit emerge in their place, for Spirit's language is love-based.
Negative thoughts drown it out, even though it is all around us
and within us.

Spirit speaks to us through our thoughts, intuition, experiences, and feelings, and even through the words of other people.
Yet we rarely hear these blessings. To do so, we must learn to be
quiet and listen, and to cease intruding our own loud voice in their
place. Spirit's voice exists beneath all the ego thoughts that drown
it out. We are not alone. Learn to still your own inner voice, and
you will realize that a powerful Guide has entered your life. Spirit
can show us which way to go, help us with major life decisions,
and teach us how to understand the lessons we came to earth to
learn.

Spirit can also speak to us through other people, even when
they are not trying to act as a channel for Spirit's voice. As you
stop judging what is being said, you will realize that sometimes
the words that another person is speaking are not coming from
their ego, but from Spirit. They answer your needs and questions. Learn to listen to the voice of Spirit, which speaks through

the world and other people, and you will receive a great gift: the counsel of the Source of all life.

Forgiveness is the way to open yourself to the type of deep peace that is necessary for you to begin hearing the voice of Spirit, whether it is coming to you through your own thoughts or another's voice. Tune in to Spirit's guidance by tuning in to the spirit of forgiveness. Whenever you need guidance, stop and listen to what those around you are telling you, as well as to your own thoughts that are grounded in gentleness. You will catch hints about yourself, the direction in which you need to head in life, the lessons you need to learn. We can hear many of the answers we are seeking through the art of inner stillness and quiet listening. Just be still, ground your mind in silence, step back, and listen. What message does Spirit have for you today?

Health and Healing

The body extends from the mind, the mind from core self, core self from Spirit. To heal, it is necessary to reopen the energy channel between body and Spirit, which has become misaligned, so that the creative, healing energy of Spirit can be received on all levels.

At conception, the body explodes with life, grows, and flourishes. Life and health, not sickness, are what is natural. Life continuously expands outward from its center in a never-ending unfolding loop. This may be difficult to understand in linear terms, but you can see the evidence everywhere. We live in a universe of life, energy, and light. Look across the earth and see for yourself. Wherever life *can* arise, it *does*. Grass grows through concrete. Plants, fish, and bacteria thrive near geothermic vents in the sea floor, where they have somehow managed to adapt to the crushing pressures at the bottom of the ocean. Stars shine their energy across a universe that seems to have no end.

Yet these are only the surface signs of life. Look through a microscope, and a universe of life appears in the world of the very tiny — from bacteria and viruses to the building blocks of matter itself, such as cells, atoms, and on and on. Where does this chain of increasingly tiny life end? Just as the gigantic world of galaxies does not appear to have an end, so it is with the invisible world that is so small, we can't even detect it without specialized scientific tools.

Wherever you look, however deeply you probe, you will find that life extends into infinity. There is no end to it, because life is eternal. And this phenomenon is not isolated to the physical world. It also has an analogous expression in the spiritual world, which we are less familiar with. Life not only extends outward into space; it also extends inward beyond the physical. Most people invest the body with faith because it is the only home they know. It is true that from our perspective, life does *appear* to begin and end here, on earth, with the body. It's important to understand, though, that the illusion of birth and death only witnesses to itself. The body's eyes are not designed to look beyond the physical world of which they are a part, so as long as we are using them exclusively, we will remain blind to what lives within us, safely beyond the physical expression and apparent deterioration of life.

The body exists in a state of seeming isolation from Spirit, and because of this, it presents us with a limited point of view. When you begin to tug at the corners and lift this veil of isolation, you start to realize that space-time and everything within it is similar to a curved loop in which aspects of creation have become trapped — like being stuck in a space-time eddy. In time we are born into a physical body, and we are suddenly cut off from the whole of creation that surrounds it, which continues on despite our own individual experiences here on earth. Imagine a swimmer who gets stuck in a whirlpool beneath a waterfall. While he tries and tries and tries again to swim free, each time the whirlpool pulls him back. Amid the turmoil beneath the waterfall, it is easy to lose track of everything else. The cascading water blinds him, and exhaustion narrows his perspective to raw, immediate survival.

In our world, everything is reversed from the way it is in Spirit. Here we believe that we live inside our bodies, trapped. Step inward and enter the realm of Spirit, however, and then look back, and you will have quite a different vantage point: we live within Spirit, and the body is the thing that is outside of us. It is like a bubble on the surface of the ocean, and we are looking up and out through the bubble from below, where we are a part of the greater sea.

It is this realization that brings healing to the body. As you free your mind from an isolated focus on the physical, you open up the body to the natural Source of healing. This highest form of communion heals because through it you are unsealing the blocks that keep you locked apart from the natural flow of life — the same expansive energy surge that brought your body into being in the first place. When you were a fetus and then an infant, your ego was not well enough formed to interfere with this growth, and so your tendency was toward health. As you grew more identified with the ego-body connection, however, this flow grew weaker, and healing was inhibited. Meditation is a step back toward this earlier, more innocent state, which is why it promotes wellness.

Everyone gets sick now and then, and over time the body does age and die. No one is immune to aging, and this book does not purport to provide a fountain of youth. There is no need for one, anyway, since life extends forever, far beyond the body. Ultimately, we must learn to come to peace with ourselves in our natural state with Spirit. I like to think of life on earth as a classroom and the body as a learning aid within the greater Earth School curriculum. The body isn't life itself, just a temporary extension of it. While we are learning, though, it can be made healthier and stronger by the way we view it, the things we use it for, and the attitudes we foster. As we learn to be more peaceful beings, the body will tend toward health. This effect follows naturally from our earlier discussion about giving and receiving being one. Quite simply, as you think healthier, happier thoughts, your body will respond accordingly.

All the many ways in which the mind affects the body make up a comprehensive and broad subject that lies beyond the scope of this book. It isn't this book's objective to prove the link between the mind and body in healing. We now have a stack of solid scientific evidence suggesting that the influence of thoughts, beliefs, and feelings on the condition of the human body is powerful indeed. Anybody is free to browse this material if they have doubts. My summary of the overall picture is simple: what you think, feel, and believe has major, scientifically observable effects on your body. Good health and healing is not a primary goal of meditation but a secondary effect. Nevertheless, physical health is an important component of peace of mind. When we feel healthy, we are happier. Pain and sickness have a negative impact on our mood, which can increase the feeling of disconnection from our Source. This is the ultimate disease. Heal this sense of separation, and you naturally heal the body.

The energy that flows from Source throughout the universe, lighting the stars and bringing life to atoms, breath to your lungs, and thoughts to your mind, is not only creative — it is reparative. When this channel is blocked, sickness becomes more likely, on every level. By reopening the energy channel between you and Source, you allow this energy to flow freely through you, and it is this that heals. Essentially, you are inviting the root creative energy of life to flow through you. That is why our curriculum has focused so intensely on the cultivation of peaceful thoughts — because such thoughts are in sync with healing Source energy. When you are sick, do not focus on healing your body. Instead, concentrate on realigning your thoughts with thoughts that reflect health. When we look beyond the body for comfort, the body itself is fortified and made well.

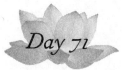

Day 71

With each quiet thought, I am blessed with the strength, vitality, and health of Spirit.

Deep meditation is an experience of unity with your core self, which is directly linked to Source. Total immersion in your core self is the ultimate healing treatment. All other types of medicine focus only on the various specific forms of illnesses instead of looking at health from a holistic approach. Because of this, they are highly limited. By turning toward Source energy for health, you ally yourself with a force so creative that it gave birth to the cosmos. Do you think a Power like this lacks the healing vitality to bring wellness to your body?

During your meditations today, try only to allow yourself to dissolve completely into Spirit, releasing all feelings of separation. Remind yourself, *"I am Spirit; Spirit is me."* For the purposes of today's exercise, imagine that there is no barrier between your mind and Spirit's mind, between your thoughts and Spirit's thoughts, between your will and Spirit's will, between your body and Spirit's body — which is not a body that is contained by walls or limitations of any kind. It is the body of all life.

You don't have to make healing happen. Just join together with the Spirit of all healing. Immerse yourself in it as if you were sinking into a pool, cleansing yourself — body, mind, and spirit — of all impurities. This analogy is not far from the truth.

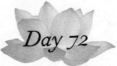

Day 72

My peace-filled thoughts are shaping a peace-filled body.

M ake your thoughts work for your health, your comfort, and your happiness. Becoming healthy has to begin with healthy thoughts, since the mind and the body are not separate. As your thoughts turn toward peace, your body *must* respond. Physical health is the equivalent of emotional health. A peaceful mind breeds a healthy body, and a healthy body supports a peaceful mind. The development of peace, then, is by far the greatest medicine. Peace doesn't pay attention to the forms of sickness but treats them by repairing their cause. Every time you choose a thought infused with compassion, the body feels a little more balanced; every time you allow a thought of forgiveness to replace a thought of anger, the body grows a little stronger; and every time you opt to look with gentleness upon a world corrupted by violence, the body feels a little bit healthier.

Day 73

I am an open channel for healing.
The rays of Source shine upon and through me,
out into the world I see and to everyone I look upon.

The miracle of healing is not limited by either time or space. The laws of our world cannot stop its passage. The healing energy of Source is a powerful jolt of divine energy that enters in the present moment and expands through you and into space-time, where it arcs out like a wave sweeping across the face of the sea. You can feel this phenomenon directly. All you need is an open mind and a willing spirit. By aligning yourself with Source, you open this channel automatically. The resulting healing wave has no beginning and no end, and the changes it can produce are not subject to any limits. It may affect your past, your present, and your future, and it may also reach out to heal people you have never even met.

Spend a few minutes reflecting on these thoughts twice today before your meditations. Remind yourself how important your practicing is, not only for you but also for a world in need of healing now. We are at a great crossroads as a people, with two distinct paths before us. One direction ushers in global peace, and the other brings disaster. The threats to our species are many, including global warming, disease, warfare, serious food and water shortages, meteor impacts, and many others. It is imperative that we begin working as a cooperative global community in order to surmount each of these crises. Yet there is great cause for hope. With each of us who chooses to become an open channel for bringing more thoughts of light into the world, we — as a race — come just a little nearer to a planetary shift in consciousness toward a more stable, peaceful earth. You can be a part of this great healing process today, with just a little practice and a little willingness. I have already made my choice for myself, as have many others. Today I invite you to decide on healing with me. To make this shift, ask yourself only one question to give your life a new direction: "Am I ready today to give in to peace and allow the healing energy of Source to move through me, to bless me, and to bring healing to all my brothers and sisters in the world?"

Day 74

Life is light, and therefore so am I.

Try imagining that at its core, all life is composed only of light. Source is light, its constant flowing out is light, and therefore so must everything that comes from it be made only of light, including thought, your body, and all things that appear to be nothing more than gross matter. We live in a universe of light, and because light is eternal, so are you. Light can never die or be made ill. It can be blocked out, as it is when you close your window blinds during the day, and it can even seem to be extinguished, as happens when you snuff out a candle's flame. However, the sun still rises each morning and even illuminates the moon by night, reminding you that although you cannot see it, it has not gone. Likewise, the core of our lives will forever abide in light, safety, unity, and wellness, even if the form changes.

While you meditate today, try to sense the core of light that comprises your life. This core makes you one with the universe and therefore protects your life forever — and you can connect with it through meditation. Try to sense its strength and feel as if you are merging into light, in both body and thought. If in previous meditations you found visualization helpful, you might even choose a simple image to help you make this connection. For instance, you might imagine a golden-hued light glowing at the center of your chest around your heart chakra, expanding to fill your body. Then try thinking for a few minutes on the idea that beneath its surface appearance, all the world of gross matter is, like you, made of light. From your body and thoughts to the bodies of all people and animals and insects, to the rocks and soil that make up the world, to the seas and lakes, to the clouds that dot the sky, to the sun, moon, and stars — all is light, and all is joined together in this brilliant, never-ending light of the universe.

Day 75

Today I am in balance with all aspects of my one self.

Sickness stems from an imbalance of energy, and wellness from bringing union to all aspects of our lives. To be perfectly well, we must feel connected to our Source; we must invest in healthy thoughts, develop healthy habits, and maintain healthy relationships. Essentially, we must strive to balance all aspects of our lives and focus them in one direction — toward healing. We can accomplish this only by relinquishing clashing goals and desires, and by wanting peace first and foremost. Health comes from peace. Joy comes from peace. Inner wealth, the only important kind, comes from peace. Seek nothing else but peace, and you are guaranteed to succeed. Seek health, then, through balance, and seek balance through peace. Recognize that more than anything else, attaining peace is the answer to all problems, including sickness. Conflict is the only problem, and peace is the solution. Even when the body is in such a state of disrepair that it cannot recover, when you are at peace, you will still find a way to view this state with equanimity. And, really, after all is said and done, what else really matters? Be at peace. Live in joy. Join in full awareness with your eternal core self.

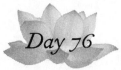

Day 76

Just as rain is made of water, I am made of Spirit.
I need only be silent and still to realize that this is true.

We are always in contact with our Source, and therefore we are always safe. We cannot truly be apart from Source, just as rain cannot be made of something other than water. Rain is water, and our souls are made of Source. How can we be separated from what we are made of? And how can Spirit be made ill?

When we grow silent enough to sense Source, we immediately recognize that we are Spirit and our bodies are only extensions of what is already within us. This thought has great healing power. First, it heals the fear that everyone, to some degree or another, suffers from on the physical plane. It's impossible to view yourself as a physical being tied to death without experiencing some fear. However, when we begin to view ourselves as anchored to a Life far greater than our individual body, we realize that we are a part of the eternal Spirit and are having a temporary experience as humans for learning purposes. This brings a sense of peace and safety with it.

Second, this realization is healing because through it we no longer isolate ourselves. When a pool of water gets cut off from its mother lake, it stagnates, it becomes imbalanced and inhospitable, and its life-sustaining nutrients are rapidly depleted. In general, ecosystems of all types are healthiest when they are inhabited by many forms of life and are not isolated and closed off from the world that surrounds them. We are just the same. The more cut off we are from other people and our Source, the worse we feel, the less energy we have, and the greater the likelihood of illness.

Reconnecting with life is the obvious solution, and we need only quiet our own internal voice so that we can better listen to the sounds of life that are all around and within us.

Practice becoming very quiet during your meditations today, and see if you can sense the Source of all life there, in the stillness beyond your thoughts, deep within you.

Day 77

Source nourishes and protects me,
offers me health when I am ill, and shelters me from all
storms of life. When I shift my awareness to Source,
I know that I am forever safe.

To continue yesterday's theme, when we see ourselves as separate from each other and Source, we belittle and weaken ourselves. Our lives seem to be those of limited organic creatures, left alone to fight against the whims of our enemies and the unforgiving, relentless turning of time — tiny, temporary specks in a hostile universe. On the other hand, by seeing our connection to all life, we realize we are joined in a union that far transcends the body, and we live in a universe that loves us and cares for us. It is our own sense of isolation that makes us feel little and weak and threatened by life.

We are not in danger, because our core self is not composed of flesh, and so it cannot be sickened. No outside force can threaten core self. We cannot starve to death, because the core self is sustained by the light of Source. We cannot be made homeless, because core self exists in a state of union with all life. We cannot grow old, because core self exists beyond time as a part of eternity. Core self lives forever and ever, beyond form, although it can express itself *in* form. This is all the body is: a creative expression, like a painting. It is not you, and you are not it. Being able to distinguish yourself from your body is a powerful lesson you would be wise to learn. It will bring you great serenity.

See yourself, instead, as you really are: a glorious living spirit, a cocreator with Source, an eternal entity living in an eternal universe. Become an active participant in your life and in the lives of all those who share this planet with you. By acknowledging the inner truth about yourself, you are becoming more natural — which is to say, more like your core self — and the more natural you are, the healthier, even in your human incarnation, you will be.

Today I view my body in a new light.
In gentleness I bless it as my sacred temple
while I am in Earth School.

Sometimes we try to punish our bodies without realizing that we are doing so. The drive to punish is hidden deep in our unconscious minds; but as we have been learning, all thoughts, unconscious or not, have power to create. Our minds were given to us by Source, the Spirit of all creation, and therefore they are naturally creative. You cannot make your mind stop creating. You can only choose *what* it will create.

So it is that we must learn to look on the body gently, use it kindly, and forgive it for the times we have misused it as a weapon. Coming to peace with your body and learning to perceive it as guilt-free is a major lesson. While you are here, your body is your temporary home and an aid designed to help you learn the sacred art of peaceful living. A big part of this lesson is coming to peace with your body. Learn to do this by respecting it and using it only for peaceful purposes. See the body as a holy temple, even if it is only a temporary one. The temple's walls are not intended to limit you or be a permanent home, but rather to provide a peaceful sanctuary where you can study, learn, and meditate. Treat your temple as you would any holy place, with reverence and care, and it will provide you with a comfortable place to abide while you are here.

Day 79

Within every passing instant, my body is reborn,
and so within every passing instant,
sickness is undone and health restored.

As we release the past and open our mind to the present, we make our body accessible to immediate health and healing. Sickness of the body can be left in the past, just as sickness of the mind can. The more willing we are to dwell only in the present moment, the easier healing becomes. An interesting notion slowly gaining scientific support is that the universe is constantly flickering in and out of existence. This constant rebirth is one of the keys to living a life that isn't plagued by disease. When you begin to think of your body as being reborn with every passing moment, you can more easily accept the idea that you are free to see your body as being reborn to health, leaving past illnesses behind as you advance into present wellness.

You accomplish this by refusing to cling to old images of your body's health. Regularly practice dwelling in the present moment, and you will begin to free your mind from the tendency to carry sickness with you from the past. Sickness always involves some preservation of past ideas about the body's condition. In other words, we think we are sick in the present only because we thought we were sick in the past. Thus we become trapped in the *idea* of sickness and carry that idea with us as we continue forward through time — like dragging an old piece of luggage with us through life. This is why when people become seriously ill, they sometimes get stuck in sickness for years, and in some cases for life. They are unable to shake the image of sickness from the past, and sickness becomes a way of life. This can be compounded when doctors tell patients that there is no cure for their ailment or that their case is "terminal." If patients believe the doctors, their own belief that the sickness will continue is reinforced.

The closer you come to dwelling in the absolute present, the closer you come to breaking this chain. Illnesses, like personality traits, are images that have been added on to core self, and so sickness is not a permanent state. We heal when we release all ancient images of sickness from our past and allow our bodies to be reborn to their natural state of health.

Free yourself from all negative past associations, and see how beautiful and strong you are in the light of the present. Each instant spent relating to the present will bring you renewed health and will free you just a little more from every negative experience that haunts you from a past that has already vanished into the swirling mists of time. The past is gone. Now you just need to learn to let it go in your mind too....

Day 80

*My body and my thoughts are one
and can never be separated.*

Try to think of the mind-body connection in this way: The thoughts you hold about your body fuse together to *become* your body. Every thought is transmitted directly to your body and affects it either positively or negatively. Your body is pure organized energy, and thought is its director. Therefore, every thought is a creator in its own right.

People sometimes ask if they should change their behavior in order to heal their body. The answer is, sometimes this is appropriate, but you must always change your thoughts first. Otherwise, no matter what you do on a physical level, your body will not respond well. No matter how great a physician's treatment plan is, no matter how powerful a medication is, no matter how minor a disease may be, no healing will occur if it goes against the mind's creative impulses. To heal, you must think healthy thoughts. Then treatments will work, and healthy behavior will likely follow. People who have forgiven their body and learned to see it in a more gentle light tend to treat it more responsibly.

Simply put, to learn how to shape your body, learn how to shape your thoughts. Become an active craftsperson, shaping your life with care, with love, with gentleness, and with conscious intent. Choose your thoughts carefully and actively, and don't allow poisonous thoughts to go unchallenged. Take a moment to consider the expression "poisonous thoughts." Every negative thought that crosses your mind, whether in regard to another person, a situation, or yourself, is poison, and it will sicken you both emotionally and physically. Learn to dislodge and replace them with thoughts of wholeness and wellness, that you may know wellness and wholeness on every level. This is the most effective path to health and healing, and it costs nothing except the relinquishment of judgment, guilt, and hatred.

Healing Relationships and Sexuality

*F*ind peace in your relationships on earth, and you will find peace in your relationship with Heaven.

It may seem strange that a book on meditation should include a chapter on relationships. Along the path to spiritual healing, however, relationships and sexuality deserve *special* attention, because our relationships tend to be *especially* screwed up! It is in our closest relationships that we tend to act out all our latent animosities and insecurities, feeding our ego a bottomless supply of negativity. Often, these relationships are where the guilt cycle is most acute and the ensuing blocks to healing most formidable. Therefore, relationships become the primary battleground where our disconnection from our core self and Source is most pronounced. In so many relationships, anger, guilt, and fear are the dominant emotions, while love is relegated to a secondary position, assuming it is present at all. Meditative practice is difficult under these circumstances for the obvious reason that turbulent feelings and thoughts directly hinder meditative states, being the exact opposite condition. For this reason, healing your relationships is an important key to learning how to meditate.

Like forgiveness, the healing of relationships is self-healing.

When you come to peace with another person, your spirit naturally reaches out and unites with that person's spirit. Through this union, the sense of separation between the two of you vanishes. To feel at one with another person heals us at a deep level. It paves the way for reconnecting with our own soul, which is the ultimate healing. As you come to peace with others and abandon the urge to use them as targets for guilt, you simultaneously release your own sense of guilt; and as a result, you come to peace with yourself.

Likewise, we often harbor much hidden guilt and shame in our sexual persona, which also may act as a block to meditation. As with any dark emotion, it is important to heal these feelings. Sexual guilt is usually directly related to the damage in our relationships, past and present, because sex is quite often used as a weapon in relationships. Also, parents sometimes unwittingly reinforce sexual guilt in their children with psychological programming that runs so deep, it can persist for a lifetime.

To heal on a sexual level, we need to stop using sex as a weapon and a reinforcement of body consciousness, and begin seeing it as an affirmation of union and love for another person. This viewpoint gradually removes the sense of guilt associated with sex. We needn't view our sexuality guiltily, but can look on it with innocent eyes. Our core self always seeks to unite with others, and sex can be one form through which this is expressed. The physical act itself does not accomplish this union. It is the *purpose* behind sex that matters. See it, like the body, as an expression of love, and it will no longer contribute to the guilt cycle. This reinterpretation of the sexual act is an important step in healing.

While this chapter is in no way intended to provide detailed instruction for healing sexuality and turning our special relationships into spiritual ones, here are some basic, essential guidelines to help you get started in the right direction:

i. *Seek only to heal yourself.* This is the first rule, and the one on which all the others are based. It can also be the most difficult to follow, but when you are able to set aside the need to try to fix others, the entire paradigm of your relationships will shift. The ego is always seeking to control and change other people, but only rarely does it accept responsibility for its own mistakes. When you follow this rule, you begin to put an end to the constant projection that makes healing impossible. By projecting the responsibility for our own feelings onto someone else, we eliminate any hope of fixing the things that are wrong inside us. When you follow rule 1 for healing relationships, you put the responsibility for your own peace and healing right where it belongs and where it can actually help — in your own hands. This guideline reflects the ancient truth that nobody can force another person to change, but people are free to choose change and healing for themselves. In fact, one *must* choose for oneself. To begin fixing your relationships, you have to withdraw your focus from trying to change others — or *any* external circumstances, for that matter — and reapply it toward yourself. Before this shift occurs, no healing is possible, because you will always blame someone else for your own distress.

2. *Don't ask, don't expect.* This rule follows naturally from rule 1. By relinquishing our expectations concerning other people's behavior, we free ourselves from the endless series of judgments and disappointments that keeps us chained to negative emotional states and experiences. This interrupts the vicious cycle of guilt and blame, freeing our relationships to heal. The rule is simple: The less you ask of others, the purer your relationships will become and the freer you will be. Just take your hands off the steering wheel and free all other people from everything you think they should do, how they should behave, who they should be. Following this guideline will

bring you incredible relief. As you release other people from your expectations, you will realize that you have also freed yourself. By setting up rules that other people must adhere to, you are building a prison out of your own expectations. It becomes up to you to monitor the people for violations and to guard them carefully to be certain that they follow your rules. Thus you become a prison guard, as much a prisoner as those you guard. Husbands, wives, and parents are particularly prone to this type of trap, but it can occur in any relationship. The instant you judge or attempt to control another person, you shackle yourself to that person — and there you will remain, imprisoned together. For a prison must have a guard, and no one will stand watch over your prisoners except you. Why should they bother, when they have so many of their own? This is the type of situation that can keep your ego happily engorged for years upon years. Interestingly, people are often surprised to find that the less they ask and expect of other people, the more that others are willing to give.

3. *Give freely and without fear.* Our third guideline for healing relationships takes things one step further. Not only should you stop asking things of others, but also it is critical to learn to give freely to them. Give of your spirit; give your energy, your attention, your love, and your time. Give, give, give, and then give some more. There is an inherent fear in each of us that as we give, we lose, but this is not the case. As you give, you will discover that you gain. We have already discussed this. Perhaps the form may change, but that is hardly important. This notion is so counterintuitive that it must be practiced to be trusted, but with experience it will prove itself to you. Try it and see. Set aside your fear of giving, and you will find a great reward. Everything you give to others, whether it is of your time or of your love, will find its way back to you,

since the law of reciprocity is fully active in all our relationships. When you relinquish your ego's demands while simultaneously giving more of yourself, those people who share your life with you will inevitably respond positively and learn the joy of giving too.

4. *Cultivate unconditional love.* This last suggestion is perhaps the most important of all. Peace is not found by imposing your will upon another, but instead through the relinquishment of judgment and the establishment of unconditional love. Defy the fear of giving love, and you will free yourself from fear. Love heals. This may sound trite and no more than a flimsy cliché with no effects in the real world of relationships, yet nothing could be further from the truth. Unconditional love heals because it is the emotional state that most closely reflects our Source, and so it invites the healing energy of Source into our relationships. As we shape our own thoughts to mirror Source, it is like opening a waterway that was dammed up. When you learn to love unconditionally, you invite the incredible healing energy of life to enter, and this energy naturally balances your relationships, essentially joining two seemingly separate individuals in one Spirit. This causes you to realize that your partner's needs are also your own, and vice versa, which leads to the related — but equally important — realization that by attacking your partner, you are really attacking yourself; by loving your partner, you are loving yourself; by freeing your partner, you are gaining your own freedom.

Applied together, the above guidelines will lead you to the awareness of your underlying unity with other people, which is what heals all relationships in the long run. The endless divisions of the world — reflected most clearly by the physical divisions between our bodies — weaken us, whereas through our unity with each other, we realize that our life is not limited to just one body. By recognizing that we are joined with another, we realize that we *must be made of Spirit*, because the life of flesh is obviously one of separation. The fact of unity proves to us that the body is not what we really are but just a passing image. Therefore, by healing our relationships, we undertake to heal at the most profound level as well — spiritually. For what is spiritual healing but the healing of the belief that we are separate from each other, our core self, and our Source?

Bonus Exercise

Start implementing these guidelines today in all your relationships. Every day should be devoted to strengthening your connection with everyone you know and everyone you meet. Begin this process by working with one of the above guidelines per week for a period of one month. For instance, begin with rule 1, "Seek only to heal yourself," and become determined to apply this to all your major relationships for a full week. Remind yourself of this goal each morning, and also remind yourself of it throughout the day whenever you are dealing with other people. Whenever you meet someone, especially if you are feeling irritated, tell yourself silently, "Let me seek only to heal myself." Use it like a mantra, repeating it as often as needed. The following week, work with rule 2, and so on.

Try to sense the ways in which these four simple guidelines make your relationships less stressful by removing your ego's agenda from them. Applying these ideas will automatically strengthen your relationships with other people, which really consist of your core self's relationship with their core self. All of our relationships should be purified in this way until interacting with others on a core level instead of an ego level becomes automatic.

Day 81

*My real relationships exist at the level of core self,
not ego. It is my core relationship with others
that brings joy to all my relationships.*

When you meet people today, look beyond their behavior, the words they speak, and the ego characteristics you see in them. Instead, direct your attention to the signs of their core self. Seek out the underlying presence of their spirit. Just as you have a core self, so do they, and each of your worldly relationships has a spiritual counterpart, or what I call a *core relationship*. This is the relationship that your core shares with their core. Relationships heal when we learn to look beyond our ego struggles with each other and perceive only our own core connection. This realization will bring you peace, and it should come as no surprise that your meditations will deepen many times over as a result.

*Unity and peace are experienced together.
The more at one I feel with others,
the more peace I will experience.*

Celebrating our differences from others marked an important stage of human evolution. This occurred only relatively recently, gathering momentum over the past century. This stage of development was important because differences have been, and frequently still are, used as weapons of attack. For example, racism derives its energy from the concept that people of a different race are inferior. Yet racism is just one example of the ego's drive to feel separate and distinct by emphasizing how it is not the same as other egos — and then to attack those differences. Any difference is suitable from an ego standpoint — race, gender, nationality, socioeconomic status, sexual preference, political affiliation, and so on. Because of this tendency, *celebrating* our differences instead of attacking them is certainly a step in the right direction. However, the next stage in our evolution goes a step further toward healing the space that appears to separate us from each other. Look carefully and you will discover that only our sense of *differentness* from others keeps us feeling separate from them. We have mentioned this point earlier, but it still needs clarification.

It is our sense of sameness with others that heals separation. Unity brings strength because it makes conflict impossible. How can a unified being conflict with itself? In your relationships, perceiving unity will do much to bring you peace. The old saying "There is strength in numbers" is truthful, but it needs one small tweak to make it more accurate: there is strength in unity, not numbers. The uniting of wills for a common cause is what lends power to any goal or situation. By joining together, we unite our power with another's, and the less sense of division there is, the more we are able to catalyze our goals.

Relationships are dynamic systems of energy exchange, and at any given instant you are using your energy to strengthen your partner or weaken them, to make them feel empowered and secure or unworthy and alone. You accomplish either of these states simply through your own focus, which alternates only between emphasizing unity or differentness. This vacillation goes on all the time, whether or not you are aware of it. The latter emphasis causes imbalances in relationships and makes them unstable. For instance, in a romantic relationship, when you make your partner feel unloved, insecure, or unappreciated, you cause them to feel unsure about the relationship. They will inevitably pull away to try to protect themselves, or they may attack you in return to try to restore their sense of self-esteem. Either way, you are not only wounding them but also weakening your own position by destabilizing the relationship of which you are an intimate part. Being in a relationship with another person is like being in a small boat together. Even when you are physically separated, your feelings and moods affect each other. And if the boat sinks, you will both go down with it. Your happiness and survival are thus tied together. So when you attack your partner, you are attacking yourself.

The closer you come to realizing unity with your partner, the more at peace the relationship will be, and the happier you will feel. This applies to all relationships, of course, not just romantic ones. Growing up in our world, which is based on differences and individuality, we are taught to either attack the differences between us or else celebrate them. Certainly, as noted, the latter advice is more positive, but an even more powerful stance is to celebrate our unity, to emphasize our similarities, and to acknowledge that our needs are firmly tied together. We live in one world, and though it may seem large, humanity's fate is interconnected in the most intimate sense. We think of our species as being composed of billions of separate individuals, but a more accurate perception is that our species is only one organism with many parts, like a plant with billions of flowers. We are humanity's flowers, and each of us depends on the whole plant's health and well-being in order to thrive and survive. If the plant dies, we all do.

You are not an island of flesh, blood, and bone with independent emotions and needs, but rather an intimate aspect of a dynamic energy play. Like it or not, the feelings of everyone in your life rub off on you because in truth we are joined as one. Their needs are your needs, and their peace is your peace. Make sure they feel loved, appreciated, and secure, and you are sure to feel loved, appreciated, and secure in return.

*I freely choose to release all people I love
from my expectations and see them as radiant beings
of light, free, happy, and at peace.*

Today, let us join together in a campaign for freedom. Let us seek to free ourselves from the delusion that by controlling other people, we will somehow find peace. Let us vow to make no demands on anyone except ourselves as we set our determination only to celebrate freedom of will for ourselves and everyone.

By trying to control others, we are heading in the direction opposite of peace, because we establish a circumstance destined to bring conflict and stress. Nobody likes to be controlled, and even if they "obey" us, they will still resent us and our relationship with them. How could peace and joy be found in such a relationship? There are far better ways to manage our relationships.

The need to control is often based on the tendency to try to make our own circumstance more stable and predictable by forcing another to adhere to our rules. For example, parents may try to control their children's choice of friends out of the fear that they might fall in with the "wrong crowd" and get into trouble, or start using drugs or having sex, and so on. This seems reasonable on the surface; however, the parents are really teaching their children that they do not trust them, that their children are not wise enough to make good decisions, and also that some people are more worthy than others. Furthermore, they are unwittingly setting up an ego need in their children, making it even more likely that they will do the very things their parents don't like. This negative parent-child dynamic weakens relationships, increases resentment, and damages children's self-esteem. It is the exact opposite of empowering them, which is the only thing we need to be concerned with if we want to protect them. Empowered people love and respect themselves and are much less likely to make poor decisions — even when you are not around to monitor their behavior.

Before you set up any expectations for someone you love, pause and remind yourself that all relationships follow the law of reciprocity, so the content of what you give to them will find its way back to you. With this in mind, ask yourself, which is the better course? To force your will on others, or to show them directly how much you trust and admire them, and to celebrate their wisdom and strength? How do you want to feel about yourself? Consider this question carefully before deciding how to treat others.

Day 84

When I seek to heal only myself,
my success is guaranteed.

None of us are perfect. That's why we are in Earth School. We all need healing. By acknowledging that you still have healing to do here, along with the fact that you can never force any other person to change, you place yourself in a position of true power. When you withdraw the energy wasted on judging others and turn that energy around to initiate personal growth, healing becomes inevitable. If you want to succeed, this is surely the way to do it.

You can't control another person's willingness to grow and evolve beyond ego. The best you can do is to provide an example of the joy that comes to those who are willing to do so. Ego loves to control, and it also loves to keep your attention focused far outside yourself and turned away from your core. It wants you to believe that the key to your own peace lies in changing other people instead of changing yourself. Look at how this ridiculous presumption makes it impossible for you to get to know your own core by keeping you constantly focused elsewhere. If you wanted to study the sky and the stars, wouldn't it make sense to begin by purchasing a telescope and taking a good look? How could you hope to learn anything about the heavens if you buried your head in the sand like an ostrich?

Release those you love from the constant need to control, direct, and judge them, and focus on your own healing instead. This way, you will be putting yourself in the captain's chair of your life by taking charge of the one thing in this world that you have power over — *yourself.*

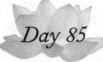

Day 85

*Unconditional love fixes all problems,
heals all relationships, and infuses my life
with a deep sense of purpose. Let me learn to love.*

I f you were to do nothing else but learn to give unconditional love to everyone you met, your life would be transformed from the inside out. The act of giving unconditional love is so powerful that it charges you with energy and infuses your life with a genuine sense of purpose. By loving another without exceptions, limitations, or conditions of any kind, you are learning to love as Source loves, and you become a channel for a type of healing that is not of this world.

The opposite of unconditional love is judgment. Judgment shuts us down from loving someone else fully by narrowing our focus to the things we don't like about the person. When we shut down from loving another, we simultaneously shut down from loving ourselves. Love is total. When you love another, you love yourself, and when you judge another, you judge yourself. We can use our mind to do only one or the other at any given instant, and we do so all the time. Our thoughts are never free from both love and judgment. As you let go of one, the other instantly fills your awareness.

What good is judgment? Has it ever given you anything of value? Did it solve your problems? Bring you joy? Infuse your life with a sense of meaning? Or did it make you feel angry, increase your sense of guilt, and bring disunity to your relationships?

You do not have to wait to learn what joy comes from releasing judgment. You may be accustomed to judgment, but you can quickly adapt to its opposite — *unconditional love* — because the feelings you will experience as you practice unconditional love are overwhelmingly compelling. Just remember, either love or judgment is with you each instant, and both have power over your relationships. If you want your relationships to be happy, you don't need to fix anything other than your own ability to love openly and unconditionally. Make it your mission to discover just what loving without exceptions means, and you may be surprised to find how powerful love is. It isn't just a sweet concept, a powerless cliché, or a lofty notion. Loving without exceptions aligns you with Source, and you will never find any experience more gratifying and empowering than that.

Day 86

Today I will start treating the people in my life
as if they really matter to me. I will show them how much
I respect and care for them through my attitudes,
my words, and my actions.

This simple change in your outlook will produce such a powerful shift that it can change the dynamic of all your relationships overnight. When you start treating the people in your life
in a way that shows them you truly care about them and let them
know through your attitudes that they matter to you, they will
feel it. Perhaps not instantly, but over time, everyone in your life
will feel the effects of this profound and fundamental shift. This
alteration in attitude will produce sweeping changes in your own
internal world as well, because as you show others that they are
worth caring about, you begin to believe that the same must be
true about yourself.

You have no need to control the people in your life, it isn't
up to you to be their guide or offer them sage advice, and you
aren't here to save them. You are here to learn your own lessons.
This is your one and only responsibility. Try looking at yourself
as a student of everyone you love and also of everyone you meet.
All relationships, no matter how casual they may seem, share the
potential to become your teachers if you are willing to set aside
your ego and accept your role as a student of life. It is Source
that is the teacher. Whenever I meet anyone, I always attempt to
see that person as a teacher of mine, for all beings originate from
Source, and therefore all beings can potentially reveal God to me.
Learn to be grateful to everyone for what they are, and you will
be flooded with gratitude for what you are.

Day 87

In stillness, I sit. In silence, I listen. In peace, I awaken.

The universe is kind to those who live in sync with kindness. Become very quiet during your practicing today, and meditate on the sense of perfect safety, protection, and quiet kindness. Realize that you are an eternal part of an eternal universe, and dissolve into the stillness that comes with a tranquil mind. You are a pure, holy aspect of a pure, holy Spirit, and you need no other training to achieve enlightenment beyond accepting yourself as you were created. Acceptance is the key to awakening. Acceptance of what you are fundamentally, not what has been added on to what you are. Focus only on letting go of all self-made images, thoughts, and personality characteristics, and listen to the silent, still spaces between your breaths and in the tiny lulls between your thoughts. Let your sense of time vanish, let the world disappear, and release your own ego as you dive deep into your core self.

Day 88

*I will use my sexuality not as a weapon
but as a natural expression of love and affection.*

Healing our sexuality is a major step toward healing our romantic relationships, and it begins with releasing the notion that sex is a guilty, sinful act. This belief bombards us from numerous sources, including our parents, churches, sex partners, and television, and we must actively refuse to accept it. Because sex can feel very primitive, it tends to remind us of our animal roots, emphasizing the body. The ego uses this as leverage to increase our sense of distance from our spiritual core. Guilt, being the epitome of dark emotions and the foundation of the guilt cycle, is the ego's greatest energy source. If it can use sex to exacerbate your sense of guilt, it will do so at every level.

A second source of sexual guilt stems from mistakes we have made in the past. Nearly everyone is "guilty" to some degree of using sex as a weapon of attack. These may be blatant attacks, such as affairs, or less obvious forms, like making our partners feel ugly, unworthy, or ashamed of their own sexuality. Whatever the forms, when you use sex as a weapon, you will feel guilty. Sex, then, will tend to activate these old guilt feelings, and by doing so, it will make your current relationships all the rockier.

Begin to heal this sense of guilt, first of all, by seeing sex not as a sinful, animal-based act but as a natural expression of Divine love. When you are intimate with your partner, use the experience to deepen your connection with them, and to make them feel loved, beautiful, and appreciated. At its highest, sex should be not just a physical act of pleasure but also a spiritual act of bonding, which is the heart of all healthy sexual relationships.

Second, examine your own sense of guilt carefully, and if you feel guilty over past actions, make a concerted effort to heal these feelings. This is not always easy, but if you are willing to look at these ugly moments as simple mistakes that all people are bound to make, but that you are determined to learn from and not repeat, you will more readily give yourself permission to move beyond them. The way to heal errors of any kind is to begin by recognizing them; become determined not to repeat them; make amends with those you have injured, if possible; and then move forward with your life as a kinder, gentler person. Healing sexual mistakes is no different.

For some people, the act of admitting their mistakes and making amends with people they've wronged can be tremendously valuable. If there are people you've hurt badly enough that you feel the need to apologize directly to them, do it. Let them know you recognize that what you did hurt them, and apologize sincerely, without asking anything in return. This has to be an unconditional, no-strings-attached deal. Keep this exercise short and simple. Don't allow yourself to be dragged into a continuing ego exchange where guilt is reinforced and more attacks ensue. Just say you're sorry, in a meaningful way, and then move forward with your life. It's an old-school rule that Mom taught us as kids, and it still is wise advice. Whether they accept your apology is not your concern. Like you, they also have lessons in forgiveness to learn.

For today's practice, think of one person whom you felt attacked by on a sexual level, and also pick one other person whom you have similarly attacked. Imagine them both sitting before you as you meditate, and briefly consider how both the hurt you received and the hurt you gave are similar. Regardless of form, they are both expressions of the guilt we all feel over our sexual urges.

Next, think of the person who injured you, and tell them, "I understand that what you did to me was a reflection of your own pain, and I forgive you for it now so that we both can be released and find peace."

Say this several times slowly and as genuinely as possible, and imagine that they acknowledge your forgiveness. Then turn to the person you hurt by your own actions, and tell them, "I understand that what I did to you was a reflection of my own pain, and I ask you to forgive me now so that we both can be released and find peace."

Listen and hear this person tell you that they forgive you. Even if they are so angry that you know they wouldn't accept your apology in real life, a part of them is still connected with Source, and this part *does* forgive you. Their core self recognizes the gift you are offering through asking for forgiveness, and this part of them is thankful.

Finish the remainder of your meditation by sitting quietly or using whatever technique you like.

In gratitude, I spend this day,
thankful for all people who share my life,
everyone I meet, and even those I think of in passing.

Whenever you meet people, train yourself to see them in the grandest of lights. The more you view them as holy teachers, the more you will learn. The more you look on them with peace, the quieter you will become. The more gratitude you give, the more you will be prepared to receive. Because you lift them up, they will lift you.

Even the things that interfere with seeing them in light — the hurts and the trials — are lessons in peace because they provide you with the opportunity to learn and grow through forgiveness. Be grateful even for the trials, then. Each time you let forgiveness replace a grievance, you brighten your heart and bring yourself one step closer to Source, one step nearer to perfect peace.

By searching out the greatness in others, through all circumstances, you will begin to awaken to the greatness that is a part of you as well. This greatness comes from the Spirit in us, of which each of us is an indispensable part. You can never be replaced. Each of us is a unique, powerful, and highly creative being. Some people believe in angels, but few of us realize that we are all angels. Think about that. You are an angel of Heaven, and you are literally surrounded by other angels! They may be angels who are learning to remember their identity, but even in this you can be of service. You become of service by seeking out the glory and power that are locked inside them, hidden even from their own view. Lift them up and remind them who they are, for they are no ordinary beings. Neither are you. But you must choose carefully how you will treat them, or else you will fail to remember your own power and glory.

By being grateful to everyone you meet, you begin the process of turning Earth into Heaven. Gratitude is a mighty spiritual teacher, for it can show you how great you can be too. Instead of judging others, begin searching out those characteristics in them that you wish to cultivate in yourself. Always look for the good in others, and you will find it both in them *and in yourself.*

Try to remember to thank everyone you meet today, silently in your own mind. Don't allow judgment to trick you into becoming blind to the greatness that surrounds you. These people are more than just your companions; they are all great spiritual teachers — and so are you.

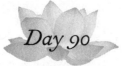

Day 90

*Love is my companion today, keeping me safe,
sheltering me from sorrow, and guiding my footsteps
along the path to perfect peace.*

Our focus today will be on trying to sense the strength and peace that come from cultivating unconditional love — not as a nice idea, but as a force with real effects in our lives. Some people believe that love is just a feeling, but true love is a dynamic energy that derives its power from Source. By *true love*, I do not mean the destructive type of "love" that is found in violent, obsessive, and codependent relationships. Just as forgiveness has both true and false forms, so does love. True love is unconditional, pure, and free from ego. It brings you a sense of harmony, quiet, and peace. Another important characteristic of true love is the feeling of freedom that comes from it. True love does not seek to control, suppress, or stifle, but to liberate and bless others.

One could not ask for a more beautiful and faithful companion through life than true love. Learn to cultivate unconditional love for everyone. If you were to do nothing else with your life but focus on this simple goal, you would become one of the most powerful human beings who ever lived. When you feel the strength that comes from unconditional love, your life will be so transformed that you will realize the path of love is the key to a deep happiness, sense of safety, and inner guidance you never dreamed could be possible in this chaotic world.

Never go anywhere without love in your heart, or else no matter where you go, the world will seem empty or, even worse, dark and dangerous. Love will soothe your memories of pain, wrap your future in peace, and paint your present with its warmth. Everything you look upon through the lens of love will seem different, new, and bright with life.

I realize that all this may sound like an exaggeration, but love does not ask belief of anyone. It only asks that you welcome it into your life, despite your doubts and uncertainty. What you then experience will be convincing indeed. Use today's mantra to begin opening up and welcoming true love into your life, and try to sense the energy of love within you. Learn to give and receive unconditional love, and watch the world transform before your open eyes.

Developing a Daily Practice

*D*evote every day to conscious living, and every day will be rich with discovery, adventure, and passion.

Learning how to meditate and sticking to a regular practice are two distinct stages of the meditative journey, each requiring different tactics. If you were meditating for some time before you started this book, you no doubt already know this. If you are new to meditation, however, you should keep certain things in mind as you continue.

The resistance to meditative practice that we spoke of before is not limited to beginners. It can persist for some time in varying forms; and it may disappear only to crop up again at a later date. Be alert for the signs of resistance you will have to confront as your practice deepens. This resistance can come in both physical and emotional forms, and as we have discussed, there are many of these. The bottom line is, *anything* that interferes with your practice should be considered a form of resistance and is best addressed forthrightly.

Because meditation challenges us at a deep, intrapersonal level and is such a direct shift toward peace, expect to be challenged by the Wolf of Darkness as you continue your journey, and become determined now not to allow yourself to be discouraged.

The Wolf of Darkness feeds on negative feelings, and by meditating regularly, you are starving this destructive force. Also bear in mind that if meditation weren't challenging, how much would you expect to get from it? Isn't it true that the most rewarding things in life are often those that challenge us the most? In fact, if you don't earn something, you will never truly understand its value. Frequently we gauge the worth of something by how much effort or money it costs us. Meditation is no different.

As you advance, don't try to evaluate your progress each day. This is like trying to record a child's growth through daily measurements. Day to day, you won't be able to make out much of a difference. Practice for six months or even a year, and then look back and measure your growth. The peace of meditation is cumulative. It will continue to grow the more you invest in it, and over time you will begin to see exponential leaps.

So the first step you need to take toward building a regular practice is to resolve firmly to practice no matter what for a predetermined period of time. No matter how you feel each day, no matter how busy you are, no matter if you feel as though you are getting nowhere, no matter what the Wolf of Darkness tells you, you sit down every day at your appointed time and you do your dharma. Just like exercise, meditation doesn't always produce instant results, but you do it anyway because you know it's good for you. Also like exercise, it may not always feel 100 percent pleasant when you're doing it. You may have to force yourself to take the time until you feel your momentum kicking in and carrying you forward. This does happen, and it happens faster for some people than for others.

A big part of what adds to the growing momentum of meditative practice is your own commitment to it. If you are uncertain and wishy-washy, your progress will be hindered. The bottom line is, the more you put into meditation, the more likely you will be to develop a lasting meditative practice that will grow richer and more joyful over time. Meditation can be a life-changing practice, and it is not only about the practice itself. It is about living a more conscious, vibrant life. It is about personal empowerment, healing relationships, and coming to peace with every facet of our own personal existence, whether on the ego level, on the physical level, or in our own core self.

Feeding Your Practice

While the most important thing for developing a successful ongoing meditative practice is to do it regularly, there are other ways of supporting your practice that you might find of use. The meditative path can feel like a lonely one at times, and so it helps to stay connected with the greater meditative community. Doing so helps in a couple of major ways. First, you can get much advice from others who, like you, have also chosen the meditative path. This can be helpful for obvious reasons. You may also benefit from the simple feeling of support. Human beings are pack animals at our core, and we gather strength and comfort from companionship, even if that company is not a direct relationship. Connecting with others via the Internet or books can be helpful in this sense.

Books, such as this one, can help keep you focused and expand your understanding. While meditation is an experience, supplementing it with book learning is often helpful. Setting aside some time for theoretical study will reinforce your experiences and may provide you with insights into the process and practice of meditation that you would otherwise overlook, or at least take much longer to figure out on your own. I encourage you to pick up other books on the topic and related subjects. At some point, it might also be helpful for you to reread this book, working your way through the daily lessons once again. Sometimes important lessons are not processed the first time through, and you may gain new insights from the same material as your experience with meditation grows.

I have also developed a *free newsletter*, which is available by email. It includes quick tips, articles, product reviews, and listings of my upcoming workshops. Visit my website, TobinBlake.com, to sign up for it.

Another good resource is *meditation groups, centers, and workshops*, where you can meet like-minded seekers and instructors and participate in group meditations. In addition to providing you with advice, groups have the benefit of offering a more direct line of support. Meeting with other practitioners can reinforce your commitment to meditation. You may even develop valuable friendships in the process, and becoming friends with other people who meditate will encourage you to continue your practice — a gift that can't be overestimated.

My only word of caution regarding meditation groups is that there are a great many teachings on this subject, and a small number of them do more harm than good. Ideally, such groups should inspire you and elicit positive feelings. The most positive paths are those that celebrate free will, not control over others. It is through your own free will that you will progress in your dharma. Your meditations will deepen and grow increasingly enchanting because you find joy in them, not because you've been forced or pressured. This is a path of freedom.

There are lots of other possibilities for expanding and supporting your practice. For example, you may wish to create a special *meditation space* in your home, although this is by no means required. Some people, though, do find it useful and inspiring to have a space decorated with images and other items that foster a sense of equanimity and inner quiet, such as pictures or small statues of enlightened beings, pillows, candles, and incense. Most of these items are available online or through meditation supply stores and local spiritual and Buddhist centers. *Music* especially designed to accompany meditation can certainly enhance your practice, providing a new dimension to your experiences. If you are struggling with your practice and find it difficult to just sit down and get to it, I strongly encourage you to sample music that helps you to relax and inspires you. You can also use *guided meditations* for this same purpose, in either video or audio versions. Check my website for links to YouTube videos I have produced to enrich your meditative experience.

The bottom line is, make meditation an important aspect of your daily life, and look for ways to feed your practice. Stay involved and connect with others. Read some books, go to an open meditation at your local dharma center, attend a workshop, buy some music, decorate a small space in your house exclusively for meditation. Do whatever makes your experience feel richer and keeps you at it day to day.

Meditation is an ever-changing path that winds through many different landscapes and produces a variety of experiences. I can tell you firsthand, it is a beautiful path unlike any other. The path can be exhilarating at times, but it can also feel boring and stagnant if you are just going through the motions. Don't let yourself get stuck. Challenge yourself and stay focused on taking your meditative practice to the next level — gradually but consistently. And by all means, when you do get stuck, reach out. There's a whole wide meditative world out there, bursting with wisdom and energy that you can benefit from.

Day 91

There are only two paths through each day I travel —
the way of fear and the way of love. Today I choose love.

For the final ten days of our journey together, we are going to review some of the major lessons we have covered and see how they tie together. Today's thought simplifies the complexity that often clouds our path through life. It is such an important concept that I urge you to remind yourself of it every day. It is easy to become overwhelmed with life's complexities when we are not living consciously. To live consciously means you are actively shaping your life, choosing your thoughts and emotions, and taking responsibility for your own decisions. When you do so, you become commander of your experiences instead of merely reacting to the random happenings that life throws your way.

The best way to begin this process is to decide each day which path you will follow. There are really only two pathways through this world, and each one will lead you through two distinct and completely opposite experiences. If you look carefully, you will notice that everything you think and feel stems from one of two primary human emotions, fear and love. These two faces of emotion are our primary guides through life.

Think of fear and love as tour guides who describe everything you see and experience, as well as everyone you meet. The voice of fear *always* speaks negatively and devises the worst possible interpretations. Don't be mistaken. This guide is not faithful, although it is consistent. It speaks negatively not only about others but about you as well. It is constantly afraid of sickness, always depressed, terrified of betrayal and abandonment, anxious to a fault, and highly judgmental. Or, in contrast, it may try to cover up its fears with a false show of bravado or superiority. We've all met people like this, and most of us have even played this role now and then. False power and false pride are just the flip side of the face of fear. You can identify this less obvious state of fear by learning what authentic joy feels like. False pride is never accompanied by the type of deep and lasting joy that comes from walking with love. Whenever you find yourself experiencing negative feelings in any form instead of joy, you can be sure you are listening to the guide of fear.

The voice of love is the polar opposite in every way. It speaks for peace, health, and happiness — not only for you but for everyone. It doesn't judge others, but forgives mistakes actively. The voice of love reminds you that you are not alone in the universe, you are not in danger, and you have nothing to fear from the future, because you are an immortal part of Spirit. It inspires a sense of safety and peace, and when problems do arise in your life — which they will! — the voice of love seeks to heal them instead of condemning and punishing.

Both of these guides speak to you through your thoughts and feelings. They are the two voices inside your head — the Wolf of Darkness and the Wolf of Light. If you want to know which wolf you are feeding at any given time, or regarding any particular circumstance or person, all you need to do is stop and listen closely to your feelings. How do you feel? Are you at peace? Happy? Are your thoughts reflective of quietness and certainty? Are you focused on healing and fixing problems and relationships? Or are you stuck in fear-based thoughts, uncertainty, judgment, guilt, depression, and sorrow?

Be honest with yourself, but when you catch yourself listening to the voice of fear, don't punish yourself. This is just more of the same negative thinking, only flipped around and redirected toward you. Instead, clearly recognize that you made a mistake and it is time to pause and reboot. You want to be at peace, you want happiness, you want to live a meaningful life, and the only way to do so is to listen to the guide for love.

Meditation is your best resource for accomplishing this. Memorize today's thought so that you will be able to use it anytime you find yourself following the wrong guide. All you need to do is close your eyes and relax into a brief meditation: spend just a few minutes repeating today's idea until it becomes your dominant thought, which means you have released judgment and fear.

The guide for fear can be persistent, but with practice you will begin to learn that you have the power to silence it and invite the guide for love to teach you instead. Sit down now and firmly set your intention to begin this new way of living today. You can do it. Once you have made up your mind to follow the path of love, there is no force in the universe powerful enough to stop you. That's how powerful your will becomes when it is united with your core self!

Day 92

I am not alone. I am one with my Source,
with everyone I love, and with all life.

You have a greater body than just the little physical one you are aware of. You share the body of Spirit, along with every other living creature in the universe and beyond. Every thought you hold that makes you feel better or worse than other people, or makes you feel different in any way, exacerbates the feeling of being alone and abandoned by this greater Body. By increasing your sense of separation from others, such thoughts also separate you from your spirit body, your core self. This adds to your sense of vulnerability and weakness. Separation thoughts may make you feel strong on the surface, but this is nothing more than an illusion of strength. Whenever you add energy to thoughts of division, you are increasing your sense that you are nothing more than a physical entity, which is necessarily bound to decay. This is an inherently fearful condition. By embracing your unity with the whole of creation, on the other hand, you will begin to realize what core self is — not as an idea but as a reality. Your life is not one of flesh and bone but one of immortal Spirit, and your spirit lives safely beyond the world you view with your eyes and touch with your hands. Your core self is the self inside you that is still connected to Spirit. Don't disconnect yourself from it by keeping yourself disconnected from other people, because if you do, you will experience fear. This is a simple law of thought, which most people don't even know exists. To come to peace, you will need to be more than just aware of it. You will need to root out all thoughts that make you feel different from others and work at healing them. The work is not always easy, but allowing thoughts of separation to fester unconsciously is far more painful.

You don't want to feel alone and isolated. There is great peace in realizing your unity with life. Not with other egos, but with Spirit. The only way to realize this is to release your judgment. Judgment — good or bad — is the mental device that keeps separation going. Instead, seek only a sense of unity with others. Do not think of them as better or worse than you, but try instead to think that each of us is a spirit in motion, with unique lessons to learn on this earth and also unique gifts to bestow. Others' gifts are no greater or less than yours, and their lessons vary only in form. Differences fade and vanish as you quiet your mind, until you realize that all life stems from one Source, and that one Source is a part of everyone.

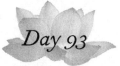

Day 93

*Nothing can harm or attack Spirit in any way,
and I am Spirit.*

Today's review flows naturally from yesterday's idea. We are safe in Spirit, so it is to Spirit that we must appeal for our stability. Spirit is our protector, provider, and comforter. We cannot look for safety and security in the world because the world is unstable, and even the earth itself will not last forever. How can you feel safe if this is your reality? Only Spirit is eternal. Therefore, if we want to feel safe and secure, which is the only state in which genuine, lasting peace can be possible, we must divest our interests in the physical and reinvest them in the spiritual.

On a physical level, of course, it is true that we can be hurt, but when we dive beneath the world of form and into the great body of Spirit, we can clearly see that we are safe from all harm. The realization that you are Spirit, and are therefore immune to all forms of injury, also justifies forgiveness. When you realize that you are safe, you can more easily see beyond attack and forgive it. In any situation in which you are angry or hurt, let your goal shift from engaging in attack, defense, and judgment to healing the relationship and fixing the problem. Embraced with total devotion, this shift in your aim alone can be enough to show you that the reverse of attack — *love* — is a far more powerful ally, because by aligning yourself with love, you are aligning yourself with the only power in the universe that is eternal.

Day 94

I am not my body, beliefs, or feelings.
I am not the roles I play in this world.
I am core self, spirit, and pure joy.

Just as our real lives cannot be threatened by anything physical, we need not seek to defend any of the intangible elements that we believe make up our personality. Like all people, you no doubt have many beliefs and values, and you play a number of different roles in this world. When you identify your existence as being dependent on principles and roles, you weaken yourself and make yourself vulnerable. This is exactly what happened when the stock market crashed in 1929. Many investors had bound their ego identities so tightly to their money that when the market collapsed, their egos went with it, and some committed suicide. This is an extreme example of how vulnerable you can become by identifying *who you are* with things that are bound to change and are easily threatened. Less extreme examples of this same principle can be seen everywhere. For instance, people who identify heavily with their career are often emotionally devastated when they lose their job, and not just because of the financial strain. Their very sense of *identity* is threatened. Similarly, parents who wrap up their sense of self with their role as a father or mother often suffer greatly when their children grow up and move away to college or get married.

Keep your identification with all such roles limited and light. Doing so will strengthen you and reduce any defensiveness and sense of threat. You will feel less vulnerable, and as a result, you will learn faster. You are not any of the roles you play in this world. The more thoroughly you realize this, the safer and more secure you will become. Identify instead with your core self, and you will gain a genuine and lasting sense of power and protection, because core self cannot be threatened and therefore requires no defense. Unlike the stock market, core self will never crash.

Day 95

*I can find happiness today, right now,
by choosing to harbor only loving thoughts.*

Today's mantra is a thought with great power. It holds the key to finding immediate happiness, no matter what you are dealing with. To know yourself as spirit, you must learn to embrace only thoughts of love, because Spirit is love. Anger, guilt, and fear will always block your awareness of core self and Source, and as a result, they will remove all hope of lasting happiness from your life. Our sense of completion comes from knowing, in full awareness, what we really are beyond our human form. Meditation makes this possible, but all negative thoughts and emotions must be healed in order for you to experience the deep peace that comes from this revelation. This is why it is essential to work diligently at reprogramming the waterfall of thought. Do not forget that your thoughts operate day and night in the background of your mind, and they will shape your life, whether or not you are aware that they are doing so.

This process of reprogramming involves a couple of important steps. First, regular meditation is essential because it creates a space of peace within you and helps you to become more aware of negative thought patterns and old unhealed grievances. In other words, it shows you both what needs to be healed and the rewards of healing. You need to heal old wounds and judgments. The result of doing so is profound peace.

Make building this space of peace a major life goal. There is nothing in this world you can do to evolve more rapidly into a conscious being than to meditate regularly.

The second important element of the process of reprogramming involves actively seeking to replace anger and judgment with forgiveness and understanding, and in general developing a peaceful worldview. Since the lessons of the Wolf of Darkness run deep, it is important that you dedicate yourself each day to undoing the negative inner dialogue that keeps you trapped in the guilt cycle.

Changing your thoughts can also have positive effects on your body, because the body is a direct extension of the mind. Try thinking of the body not as flesh and bone but as a vessel that is composed of thought and light. If this is true, doesn't it make a great deal of sense that if your mind is dominated by negative thoughts, your body will tend toward negative states? Likewise, it is easy to see how when you shift your thought patterns in a positive direction, your body will be just as likely to reflect these healthier thoughts. The body itself is neutral. It can only reflect your dominant thought pattern. This is just one more good reason to make big changes in the way you think.

To stay healthy, challenge all negative thoughts that occur to you, and reject them. This practice is essential to health on every level. Feed your mind only thoughts that are nutritious and balanced, and both your body and your mind will respond with renewed vitality.

Day 96

*I experience only what I feel for others,
which is why I choose to harbor only thoughts of purity
and blessings for everyone I meet.*

Ridding yourself of dark emotions ultimately requires you to forgive your sense of guilt. This idea has appeared in many ways in the book because it is your golden key to peace. If you were to grasp only this lesson and apply it, you wouldn't need any of the others. Forgiveness of personal guilt, or *self-forgiveness*, is an essential step in the process of coming to peace. The trick is, it is impossible to be free of guilt while you are still projecting it toward other people through anger, judgment, and attack. As you learn to forgive other people for their mistakes, however, your forgiveness automatically transfers back to you via the law of reciprocity. This is how you heal guilt and open to deep meditative states. In this sense, forgiveness can rightly be considered an advanced meditation practice. There is no mantra or special breathing technique that will increase the depth of your meditative practice the way forgiveness will.

Most effective meditation techniques merely help instill a sense of peace, thus alleviating some of the fear and guilt that is latent in the human psyche. The more peaceful and quiet your thoughts, the closer you come to core self. When you are focusing on a peaceful image during meditation, such as in visualization, the image is there only to help you find the key to inner quietude and thus sink more deeply into your practice. However, by supplementing mere techniques with much more profound exercises such as forgiveness, you will greatly amplify your practice. Do not underestimate the effects of forgiveness and nonjudgment. If you were to focus on nothing besides learning how not to judge, meditation would become so natural that you would no longer need any techniques at all. Every day should be devoted to learning the great art of forgiveness. This is the one activity you can do in this world that will ensure a life filled with meaning, authentic development, and joy. The more deeply you go into the ways of forgiveness, the more incredible your journey will become. Wouldn't you like to live a life in which every day was a magical adventure of learning and discovery? This is the path that forgiveness offers.

Day 97

*In this present moment, I am free of the past
and free of the future, and I find myself at peace
in the stillness and silence of my core self.*

True peace of mind always involves releasing thoughts of the past and concerns about the future. The mystical moment is the deepest experience of the present, which forms a doorway that leads us beyond time. To enter the mystical moment, you must stop doing and also stop judging, and *just be*. By relating directly to the present instead of focusing on thoughts of the past or future, you get a feeling of what you are outside time's walls. Your core self has always been, and as you realize that you are one with it, you will know that *you* have always been too. Your birth into the world did not mark your birth into life. You existed before your body's life, and you will continue your journey even after your body is gone. This realization is available to you in any instant, because the present moment must be — by definition — forever present.

Learn to turn to it in any instance or circumstance in which you need guidance or become tired of suffering and want peace instead. Every time you turn to it by releasing your projections through time, you will be pleasantly surprised by how powerful it can be — how it reshapes your mind and heals your feelings. The power of the present moment is always with you, all the time, and it goes with you everywhere. The present is the only time there is. By becoming present, you are thus leaving fantasy behind and communing with reality.

Day 98

*Spirit is always with me, and speaks to me
through everything I see and everyone I meet.
I need only learn to be still and listen.*

We are not alone in this world. Within each of us is a Great
Teacher who helps us to learn all the lessons we came to
Earth School to learn. For every painful experience, this Teacher
extends a lesson in healing. To be able to hear this Teacher, though,
we must learn to be very quiet and listen, for this Teacher, being
the Teacher of gentleness, speaks softly, and our own voice can
easily drown it out.

When we do learn to be quiet, Spirit will speak to us through
our own thoughts, as well as through other people and even random "coincidences." There are no big coincidences in life. If you
catch yourself thinking, "What a strange coincidence!" it probably wasn't a coincidence at all, but the Great Teacher of Earth
School pointing out some lesson you needed to learn or a new direction your life needed to take. Open your ears, open your eyes,
stop judging, and start paying attention to the world both within
you and without. Stop, listen, and become present and alert. What
is Spirit trying to tell you today? What path is Spirit pointing out
to you? Whom would Spirit have you meet, and what should you
say and do? What lessons are you meant to teach and learn today?

Become a conscious student of life instead of a passive pas-
senger. All lessons of Spirit can bring us to ever deepening states
of peace, self-realization, and the awareness that the universe we
live in is filled with Life — Life that is intelligent, aware, and
highly active in our own lives. Spirit knows you well, understands

what lessons you need to learn in order to heal, and can show you which path will lead you to happiness and peace. In fact, Spirit knows you far better than you know yourself because its vision is unlimited. Spirit guides us truly all the time, every day, but how can we hear when our minds are filled with chaos? Learn to be still and listen, and you will clear a space in your mind to receive guidance that is wise beyond the counsel and teachers of this world. It is only this guidance that will bring you the deep rest your soul craves.

Day 99

Deep within me is my homeland.
I need do nothing to return home but free my mind,
let go, and sink into the quiet space within.

Our real home is not in the world outside of us, but rather the one inside of us. We are unaware of this sacred inner world only because we have become totally focused on the outside world, and our anger, guilt, and fear stop us from looking deeply within. Seeing beyond the veil of guilt and reconnecting to our homeland is the great gift of meditation and why regular practice is such an important part of living a balanced, healthy life. By turning within, closing your eyes to the world, and exploring inner space, you are attempting to reach your original self. This contact not only heals us on the inside, but also can cause dramatic shifts in the way we perceive the world and our relationships. Each time you meditate, you are cleansed in Spirit, renewed in both body and soul, and purified. Each time you meditate, your life shifts just a little more in a positive direction. Each time you meditate, you come away from your practice more balanced, clearer, and stronger. Each time you meditate, you go home for a little while.

From this day forward, I abide in peace. I set aside all negative thoughts and accept into my mind only thoughts that lend themselves to my happiness and quietness of thought. From this day forward, I abide in peace.

While meditation is most effective when practiced twice a day, you shouldn't use a lack of time as an excuse not to practice at all. If you can find time to meditate only once a day, or even just a few times a week, it is certainly better than nothing. Just be certain to supplement your meditations with as many thoughts of peace as possible, which will add their energy to your efforts.

To reiterate, I usually recommend that new students meditate between five and twenty minutes at a time for the first year or so. After that, if you are feeling comfortable with longer meditations and your schedule allows for extended practice, you may wish to increase your regular sessions to about half an hour.

After having experimented over the past hundred days, you should have a pretty good feel for which forms suit you — whether meditation with a mantra, visualization, a chakra meditation, or just sitting. Set a time frame in advance — a few months to a year — during which you will practice with one form only; afterward, you can look back and decide if you would like to switch forms or continue your practice as is. Sticking to a single practice for an extended period has its benefits, as does changing things up periodically.

Remember, meditation is a simple, humble path, and so it is

that humble techniques often work best. Don't be conned into believing there is some mysterious, magical technique. Meditation is real work, work that is about coming to peace in a world of war, and that means tackling your own inner demons. This should always be your primary focus, not trying to change the world or fix other people. For if you achieve inner peace, you will see everything through that filter. Master your mind, and you master the world.

Epilogue: Connecting with Your Inner Teacher

Peace can never be found by making changes in the outside circumstances of your life, but only through the choices you make, moment to moment.

I have a confession to make. I do not really consider myself a meditation teacher, for *meditation is the Teacher*. Meditation is a great and ancient spiritual Teacher that has been a part of human life since the beginning of recorded history. The Hindus were using it thirty-five hundred years ago, and there is evidence that its use began long before that. If you do not like the word *spiritual*, you may substitute the word *life*. In this context, they mean the same thing. Meditation is a great *life Teacher*, and it is always accepting new students. Therefore, my role in this process is less a teacher's and more a host's. I can only introduce you to my Teacher. It is the Teacher's job to take you under its wing, if you are a willing student. Meditation can accept only willing students, for it is a gentle Teacher, being a Teacher of gentleness itself. If, however, you are seeking a Teacher who can fill your life with meaning and show you the joy of living, you have met your match. Just because this ancient Teacher is gentle does not mean it lacks the ability to change lives.

And what is the path that meditation guides you along? There are a couple of important things to bear in mind as you continue. First, meditation's path is an internal one. It doesn't ask you to make big external changes, but rather quiet inner shifts in the way you think. Learning its lessons involves learning how to reshape your thinking away from blame and toward love. All of meditation's teachings are geared toward this shift in thought.

Second, meditation doesn't ask much. Give it just a little attention and a little love each day, and your rewards will be profound. The only thing that will seriously threaten your progress is if you actively resist or stop practicing entirely. To avoid this, take meditation seriously, and also take the process of reprogramming seriously. Never make big decisions without meditating on them first and asking explicitly for guidance. This means you ask and then you *listen*. Learn to be quiet and hear your Teacher's voice. Meditation is not just a passive process; it is an active Teacher with the ability to guide and advise you in *all* matters. Meditation's guidance comes directly from Source.

I do not believe in coincidences, and so it is that I do not believe you have read this book by accident. Earth is a school, and until we begin taking the lessons we came here to learn as our ultimate responsibility, our progress in the curriculum will be slow and our path will be rocky. You have reached an advanced stage in this process. I know this is true because meditation is an advanced course in Earth School. Practicing regularly will speed up your progress exponentially. Keep in mind that meditation's guidance does not end when you are done sitting for your morning practice. This Teacher will accompany you through each day and provide you with peace in all your interactions if only you invite it to. Don't limit its guidance.

Spend time in your Teacher's presence every day, and make a habit of taking some thought of peace with you as a companion — like those presented in this book. You can find such thoughts anywhere when you start paying attention and looking for them — in song lyrics, poetry, books, movies, magazines, television shows; from other people; and even in your own mind. The more thoughts of peace you feed your mind each day, the more empowered you will become. Each thought of peace you hold and repeat through the day is like a seed that will germinate and one day sprout to provide you rich sustenance. Repetition of thought is a powerful thing. It is so powerful, in fact, that it can destroy or restore your life, throw you into the depths of depression or lighten your mind with joy — depending on the nature of the thoughts. Use that power to your advantage to free yourself from pain and build a life that inspires you and everyone around you. Never take your thoughts for granted, but become the captain of your life by taking charge of them. You do this not through long and hard practice but by making gentle yet consistent effort each and every day.

Listen to your feelings, and use them as a guide to steer you toward thoughts that are in line with joy and quietness. Pay careful attention to your thoughts. Negative thinking patterns come in many forms. When you catch yourself thinking negative thoughts — whether about another person or yourself — remind yourself that this is a pattern you have decided to let go of, and then intentionally shift your thoughts toward empowering ones. If the voice in your head is telling you things like "I am not good enough, I am not smart enough, nothing ever works out for me, I can't do this," you can be sure that you are listening to the Wolf of Darkness. Pause long enough to reverse this and begin thinking opposite thoughts, even if you don't fully believe them at first. Say instead, "I am good enough, I am smart enough, everything works out for my own best interests, and I *can* accomplish anything I put my mind to." The same procedure should be followed when you catch yourself judging or thinking unworthy thoughts about other people.

Just as important, if you come to a place where you feel lost and without hope, learn to turn inward and become still, and focus only on reconnecting with your core self. Doing so will help solve your problems far more effectively than trying to fix them from an ego level.

The Six-Point Path

For those wanting a more structured path, the following is a six-point spiritual system that I developed over many years while working with students and dealing with my own struggle to reconnect with my core self and Source. I present it here as a final supplement for your study and consideration. You will notice that these points have already been introduced in the book, and you have been practicing them in many forms; therefore, they are presented in a very brief summary here. If you are looking for a new way of living that isn't plagued by confusion and pain but instead offers real peace, begin living your life based on these simple principles, and you will guarantee yourself rewards that exceed the ability of words to express:

1. *Meditate daily.* Actively work to build a space of balance and serenity through the regular practice of silence, stillness, and inner seeking. Meditation turns you in the direction of your true self, and so it is your most valuable tool for empowerment and personal growth.

2. *Cultivate inner peace.* Peace is the key to deep meditation, but its rewards soar well beyond meditative practice. Peace is also the key to happiness. If you want to be happy, you will need to become vigilant in your quest to develop genuine peace of mind. This process does not necessarily involve changing the external circumstances of your life, but it does require you to change hurtful and limiting thought patterns.

3. *Mind the law of reciprocity.* Use this natural cause-and-effect law to replace pain with joy, conflict with peace, and weakness with strength. As you give, you receive. Honor the power of thought.

4. *Practice present-moment awareness.* Thoughts about the past and future obliterate your awareness of the present,

which is the access point to core self. The more centered in the present you become, the closer you align with your core and the more of its energy you invite into your life. Also, pay attention to how focusing on the past breeds depression, and focusing on the future arouses anxiety. Learning to dwell in the present will free you of these negative mental states and energize your life.

5. *Heal your relationships.* Release the need to control others, learn to give instead of take, and devote yourself to loving without conditions. By healing your relationships, you will find great peace and make enormous spiritual advances.

6. *Embrace forgiveness and exercise nonjudgment.* Forgiveness heals the guilt cycle, which will free you from guilt and fear and will also alleviate the urge to attack. The release that comes from embracing forgiveness and its cousin, nonjudgment, is indescribable. True forgiveness is the most advanced of all spiritual tools. Every day should be devoted to learning and following the gentle ways of forgiveness.

A new awareness is blossoming across our planet — an awareness that we are not separate individuals with different needs, but rather that we share one life and one great need: to remember and realign with our core self and Source, to heal the damage that our egos have done to this planet and its various life forms, and to unite as one people in peace. This new awareness is a great awakening that is spreading from person to person, across every nation of the planet, like a wave across the ocean. We all must do our part.

The path of healing presented in this book and outlined above is one way for you to join this great awakening, experience it for yourself, and add your own energy to it. There are many such paths, all leading to the same realizations. Some are more direct than others; some are happier than others; some are more tranquil than others. This book suggests a way of living that combines the very best of both ancient and contemporary spiritual teachings. It is simple, easy to follow, and highly effective. For those who choose to continue, there will be many grand vistas and stunning realizations along the way, which will lead you steadily but certainly into increasing states of joy, self-discovery, and freedom. May you choose your path with wisdom and care, and may Source light your way back into peace and guide your feet so that your journey will be gentle and free from fear. *Welcome to meditation!*

Notes

Part One: Introduction

Page 8, *the brain is* physically *affected by the practice*: University of California, Los Angeles, "Meditation May Increase Gray Matter," ScienceDaily, www.sciencedaily.com/releases/2009/05/090512134655 (accessed May 25, 2011).

Page 8, *They reported significant differences in the expressions*: Jeffery A. Dusek et al., "Genomic Counter-Stress Changes Induced by the Relaxation Response," PLoS ONE 3, no. 7, e2576 (July 2008), www.plosone .org/article/info%3Adoi%2F10.1371%2Fjournal.pone.0002576.

Page 9, "*the largest increase [of stem cells] I've ever seen*": *Krista Tippet on Being*, "Stem Cells, Untold Stories," American Public Media, being .publicradio.org/programs/2009/stem-cells/ (accessed May 25, 2011).

"The Development of Peace," Day 24

Page 79, *You are going to use this person and your grievances with them in an attempt to touch, if only faintly, the release that forgiveness can bring*: Grammar buffs may notice that the use of the pronoun *them* in this sentence is incorrect, since it is a plural pronoun subbing for a singular pronoun. Every book presents unique editorial challenges, and many of the exercises in this one were especially challenging with regard to pronoun usage. After a bit of debate, we decided that in this case, and in some others that follow, it was easiest to be grammatically incorrect for the sake of clarity, consistency, and flow.

About the Author

Tobin Blake is the author of *The Power of Stillness: Learn Meditation in 30 Days*. He received his formal training in meditation and Kriya Yoga through Self-Realization Fellowship, an international organization with more than five hundred meditation centers in over fifty countries that was founded by the great Paramahansa Yogananda. He has studied many forms of meditation and has been practicing for more than twenty years. Tobin is also a longtime student of *A Course in Miracles*, a profound system of spiritual mind training that has had an impact on many thousands of people worldwide.

Tobin's short stories, nonfiction, and poetry has appeared in a number of publications, including *Surfer* magazine, and several anthologies.

Born and raised in Los Angeles, he resides in Bend, Oregon, a varied land of rivers, temperate rain forests, and frosted mountain peaks just off the eastern shoulder of the Cascade Mountains. He has two daughters.

NEW WORLD LIBRARY is dedicated to publishing books and other media that inspire and challenge us to improve the quality of our lives and the world.

We are a socially and environmentally aware company, and we strive to embody the ideals presented in our publications. We recognize that we have an ethical responsibility to our customers, our staff members, and our planet.

We serve our customers by creating the finest publications possible on personal growth, creativity, spirituality, wellness, and other areas of emerging importance. We serve New World Library employees with generous benefits, significant profit sharing, and constant encouragement to pursue their most expansive dreams.

As a member of the Green Press Initiative, we print an increasing number of books with soy-based ink on 100 percent postconsumer-waste recycled paper. Also, we power our offices with solar energy and contribute to nonprofit organizations working to make the world a better place for us all.

Our products are available
in bookstores everywhere.
For our catalog, please contact:

New World Library
14 Pamaron Way
Novato, California 94949

Phone: 415-884-2100 or 800-972-6657
Catalog requests: Ext. 50
Orders: Ext. 52
Fax: 415-884-2199
Email: escort@newworldlibrary.com

To subscribe to our electronic newsletter, visit
www.newworldlibrary.com